GLENCOE

ELECTROCARDIOGRAPHY
for Health Care Personnel

Kathryn A. Haddix R.N., M.S.
Patricia DeiTos B.S.N., B.A.

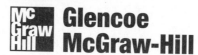

Glencoe
McGraw-Hill

New York, New York   Columbus, Ohio   Woodland Hills, California   Peoria, Illinois

Dedication

To my father, who taught me to "persevere."
—Kathryn

To my family who provided me with
love, support, and encouragement
—Patricia

Library of Congress Cataloging-in-Publication Data

Haddix, Kathryn A.
  Glencoe electrocardiography for health care personnel / Kathryn A. Haddix, Patricia DeiTos.
    p. cm.
  Includes bibliographical references and index.
  ISBN 0-07-820309-0
  1. Electrocardiography. I. Title: Electrocardiography for health care personnel. II. DeiTos, Patricia,–III. Title.

RC683.5.E5 H256 2000

00-059327

Glencoe/McGraw-Hill

A Division of The McGraw·Hill Companies

Electrocardiography for Health Care Personnel

Send all inquiries to:
Glencoe/McGraw-Hill
8787 Orion Place
Columbus, OH 43240-4027

ISBN: 0-07-820309-0

  2 3 4 5 6 7 8 9 0 079 06 05 04 03 02 01

Acknowledgments

It is a wonderful experience to see this text develop from a mere idea into what you are using today. Many individuals have spent much time and effort in providing input toward the success of this project:

- Patti DeiTos, RN, MSN, my coauthor, for all her expertise and patience in preparing Chapter 5 and the supplemental charts and materials found in the resource guide.
- James Booth, the programmer who provided the technical expertise for development of the accompanying CD-ROM.
- Beth and Pam Buckwalter, who provided much assistance throughout the project development.
- Debbie Fitzgerald, MS, RN, for her assistance and consultation with content.
- Virginia Heart Institute, including Dr. Baird and his daughter Ann Baird, who allowed us to do much of the filming and photography for the project at their facility.

Special thanks go to the reviewers who spent many hours helping us make this project complete and accurate:

Civita Allard
Mohawk Valley Community College
Utica, New York

Vicki Barclay
West Kentucky Technical College
Paducah, Kentucky

Nina Beaman
Bryant and Stratton College
Richmond, Virginia

Cheryl Bell
Sanz School
Washington, D.C.

Lucy Della Rosa
Concorde Career Institute
Lauderdale Lakes, Florida

Myrna Lanier
Tulsa Community College
Tulsa, Oklahoma

Debra Shafer
Blair College
Colorado Springs, Colorado

Preface

The field of health care is an ever-changing place. Flexibility is key to obtaining and maintaining your career. The concept of cross training, or multiskilling, although not a new one, has become the expected rather than the exception. Cross training allows you to be able to function in a variety of workplace settings doing diverse tasks. The fact that you are currently reading this book means that you are willing to acquire new skills or specialize the skills you already possess. This willingness translates into your enhanced value, job security, marketability, and mobility.

In 1994 the National Health Care Skills Standards (NHCSS) were developed by the National Consortium on Health Science and Technology Education (NCHSTE) to help serve the needs of diverse client populations, maintain quality care, and increase the efficiency of staff utilization. These standards inform current and future health care workers, employers, and educators about what skills and knowledge workers need in order to succeed. The goal of these standards is to help provide the foundation for better worker preparation and performance. This series has been written with these standards in mind. For a listing of these standards go to the NCHSTE website at www.nchste.org. All of the modules of the text include features that correlate directly with the NHCSS. The following sections describe features found within the text and CD-ROM.

TROUBLESHOOTING

The troubleshooting feature identifies problems that may arise when you are performing a procedure and provides suggested solutions. Reading these will help you answer the "What Would You Do?" questions in the Chapter Review and prepare to practice your skills in real life.

SAFETY AND INFECTION CONTROL

As a health care employee you are given the responsibility to provide safe care and prevent the spread of infection. The Safety and Infection Control feature presents special tips and techniques related to the skills taught within each module that will help you meet these responsibilities.

PATIENT EDUCATION AND COMMUNICATION

Client interaction and education and intrateam communication are integral parts of health care. You should be able to communicate effectively both orally and in writing and provide for patient education related to the procedures you will be performing. The Patient Education and Communication feature provides ways for you to perform these tasks.

LAW AND ETHICS

When working in the health care field you need to understand legal responsibilities, limitations, and the implications of your actions. You must perform duties within established ethical practices. The Law and Ethics feature provides specific information to help you gain a greater knowledge of how law and ethics relate to the performance of your duties.

Get Connected to the Web

In this technologically advanced world the Internet can be a key resource for your reference and education. Provided at the end of the Chapter Reviews are Internet sites to research and activities to complete.

Key Terms and Definitions

Each chapter begins with the identification and definition of all the key terms. On the accompanying CD-ROM the key terms and definitions are provided in audio format within each chapter and in the Glossary. You can review and listen to every key term's pronunciation and definition.

Competency Sheets

The competency checklists on CD-ROM can be used to review the skills presented and provide a check sheet for you to practice and become proficient in performing the various procedures. These competency checklists can also be used when studying or for review prior to clinical performance.

Interactive Drill, Practice, and Review CD-ROM

The CD-ROM is provided with your text to allow you to interact with and review the materials through multimedia. It is designed to complement and enhance your textbook. You can search for and listen to all of the key terms or study the competencies through interactive slide shows. Once you enter the main menu you can study each chapter. The *Law and Ethics, Providing Safety and Infection Control, Patient Education and Communication,* and *Troubleshooting* screens include critical thinking questions for you to complete, print, and check your answers. A key to your success for learning the information in this text is to study using the *INTERACTIVE QUESTIONS* provided for each chapter. They allow you to review and test your knowledge. These questions include graphics, photos, and sound that will enhance your retention of the material in an interactive way. Your score for these questions and suggested areas of improvement can be printed for you and your instructor. The Interactive CD-ROM also provides a Student Review PowerPoint Presentation for each chapter.

Instructor's Manual

Look in the Instructor's Manual for multiple resources to use while studying "ECG for Health Care Personnel." Included are PowerPoint presentations of each chapter for classroom instruction and additional presentations for student review. Many suggested classroom activities are provided that will increase the interest level and comprehension of the text/workbook material. Also, anticipatory set activities to stimulate and enhance the learning for each chapter are included. In addition, you will also find curriculum suggestions for how to use the materials based upon the length and depth of your ECG course. The interactive CD-ROM provides activities for various learning methods, and the Instructor's Manual includes instructions and suggestions for how you may want to include it in your classroom. The Instructor's Manual also includes AAMA, AMT, and SCANS correlation charts and competency checklists for the skills presented in the text/workbook.

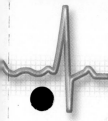

Table of Contents

Chapter 5: ECG Interpretation and Clinical Significance 72

Chapter 6: Exercise Electrocardiography 112

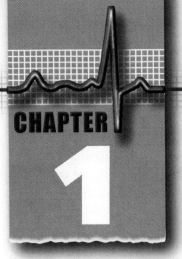

CHAPTER 1

Role of the Electrocardiographer

Objectives

Upon completion of this chapter, you should be able to:

▶ Explain what an ECG is and its importance in medicine

▶ Discuss the history of obtaining and using the ECG

▶ Describe career opportunities for an electrocardiographer

▶ List the uses of the ECG in the hospital, in the doctor's office or ambulatory clinic, or outside of a health care facility

▶ Identify the skills and knowledge needed to perform an ECG

▶ Define troubleshooting and explain its importance to you as a health care professional

Key Terms

angioplasty - Surgical repair of blood vessels.

arrhythmia - Abnormal or absence of normal heartbeat, also known as *dysrhythmia*.

cardiovascular - Related to the heart and blood vessels (veins and arteries).

Code Blue - The term used for an emergency when a person has a cardiac or respiratory arrest in a hospital or other health care facility.

coronary artery disease - Narrowing of the arteries surrounding the heart causing a reduction in the blood flow to the heart.

defibrillator - A machine that produces and sends an electrical shock to the heart that is intended to correct the electrical pattern of the heart.

electrocardiogram (ECG) - A tracing of the heart's electrical activity recorded by an electrocardiograph.

electrocardiograph - An instrument used to record the electrical activity of the heart.

electrocardiology - The study of the heart's electrical activity.

galvanometer - An instrument that measures electrical current.

hepatitis - Inflammation of the liver, usually caused by a virus.

HIV (human immunodeficiency virus) - The virus that causes AIDS (acquired immune deficiency syndrome).

Holter monitor - An instrument that records the electrical activity of the heart during a patient's normal daily activities; also known as an ambulatory monitor.

myocardial infarction (MI) (heart attack) - A blockage of one or more of the coronary arteries causing lack of oxygen to the heart and damage to the muscle tissue.

pacemaker - A cell or group of cells in the heart that affects the rate and rhythm of the heartbeat.

pacemaker (artificial) - A device, not occurring naturally in the heart, that affects the rate and rhythm of the heartbeat.

rhythm - The regularity of an occurrence such as the heartbeat.

technician - An individual who has the knowledge and skills to carry out technical procedures.

Key Terms (cont.)
technologist - An individual who specializes in a field of science.

telemetry - The transmission of data electronically to an unattached or distant location.

Introduction

The number one cause of death in America is **cardiovascular** disease. Approximately 500,000 people in this country die every year because of **coronary artery disease**—250,000 of those within an hour of initial symptoms. See Table 1-1 for information about major risk factors of heart disease. Today, more than one in five Americans suffer from some form of cardiovascular disease. You may know someone who has hypertension (high blood pressure) or other heart conditions. Maybe someone you know has had an MI (myocardial infarction, or heart attack). The **electrocardiogram** (ECG) is an important diagnostic tool used in the evaluation of cardiovascular diseases and is part of the branch of medicine known as electrocardiology. Electrocardiology is the study (*ology*) of the electrical (*electro*) activity of the heart (*cardi*). ECG is also known as EKG, which is taken from the Dutch spelling of the word "electrokardiogram." In this text, we will use the letters ECG.

There are many indications or reasons why an ECG is done. Besides diagnosing heart disease and abnormalities of the heart, ECG tracings can provide information about the heart's rate and **rhythm,** or electrical activity of the heart. An ECG may be performed for any of the following reasons:

Table 1-1 Major risk factors for heart disease

Factors that are unchangeable

- **Increasing age** - Four out of five people who die of coronary heart disease are age 65 or older. Older women who have heart attacks are twice as likely to die from them within a few weeks than men.
- **Gender** - Men are at greater risk and have heart attacks earlier in life. After menopause, the death rate for women with heart disease increases.
- **Heredity (including race)** - Children of parents with heart disease are more likely to develop it themselves. African Americans have more severe hypertension, thus increased risk for heart disease.

Factors that can be changed

- **Cigarette and tobacco smoke** - Smokers' risk of heart attack is more than twice that of nonsmokers. Chronic exposure to environmental tobacco smoke (second-hand smoke, passive smoking) may increase the risk of heart disease.
- **High blood cholesterol levels** - Increased blood cholesterol levels increase heart attack risk, especially when other risk factors such as high blood pressure and cigarette smoke are present.
- **High blood pressure** - High blood pressure increases the risk of stroke, heart attack, kidney failure, and congestive heart failure. When high blood pressure exists along with obesity, smoking, high blood cholesterol levels, or diabetes, the risk of heart attack or stroke increases several times.
- **Physical inactivity** - Lack of physical activity is a risk factor for coronary heart disease. Exercise can help control blood cholesterol, diabetes, and obesity as well as help to lower blood pressure in some people.
- **Obesity and overweight** - People who have excess body fat are more likely to develop heart disease and stroke even if they have no other risk factors.
- **Diabetes mellitus** - Even when glucose levels are under control, diabetes seriously increases the risk of heart disease and stroke.
- **Other factors** - Individual response to stress may be a contributing factor. Some scientists have noted a relationship between coronary heart disease risk and stress in a person's life, their health behaviors, and their socioeconomic status. These factors may affect established risk factors. For example, people under stress may overeat, start smoking, or smoke more than they would otherwise.

(Adapted from the American Heart Association Risk Factors for Coronary Artery Disease 1999)

- to determine how well the heart is pumping and contracting
- to check for problems with the flow of electricity through the heart
- to diagnose changes in the heart rhythm
- to check for abnormalities before surgery
- to assist in evaluating a person's health after age 40 during a complete physical exam
- to monitor or evaluate individuals with heart conditions

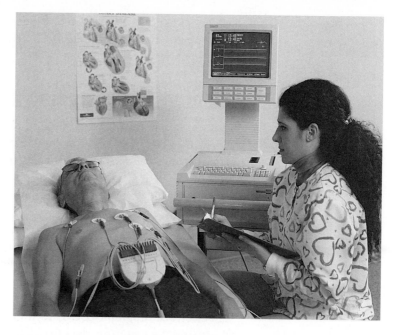

An instrument used to produce the ECG tracings, which allows the heart's electrical activity to be studied, is known as an **electrocardiograph.** The machine records the electrical activity within the heart. It is used to produce an electrical (*electro*) tracing (*graph*) of the heart (*cardio*). This tracing is known as an **electrocardiogram,** or ECG. The standard ECG machine has lead wires that are attached to a patient's chest to produce the electrical tracing (see Figure 1-1).

Figure 1-1: A 12-lead ECG machine is attached to the patient's chest, arms, and legs using electrodes and leads. It records the electrical tracing of the heart.

Performing the actual ECG procedure is not difficult; however, it must be performed competently. The tracing of the electrical current of the heart must be accurate because it is used to make decisions about a patient's care. An inaccurate tracing could result in a wrong decision about the patient's medication or treatment. These decisions could result in a negative outcome for the patient.

History of the ECG

Knowing the history of obtaining electrical tracings of the heart will help you better understand the reasons ECGs are performed and their importance in medicine. As early as 1676 scientists made the discovery that animals generate electricity. In 1887 an English physician, Dr. Augusta D. Waller (1856–1922), was the first to show that electrical currents are produced during the beating of the human heart and can be recorded. Dr. Waller was credited with having performed the first electrocardiogram on a human.

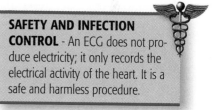

SAFETY AND INFECTION CONTROL - An ECG does not produce electricity; it only records the electrical activity of the heart. It is a safe and harmless procedure.

Wilhelm Einthoven (1860–1927), a Dutch physiologist, continued the development of the ECG. He developed the first practical **galvanometer,** an instrument used to detect electrocardiograph waves. In 1903 Einthoven invented the first electrocardiograph. Einthoven's instrument introduced the field of **electrocardiology,** and he won the Nobel Prize in physiology or medicine in 1924 for the significance of his invention.

Other scientists extended the work of Einthoven. Sir Thomas Lewis of London (1881–1945) studied how the ECG related to cardiac **arrhythmias** (abnormal heartbeats). He formed the basis for much of the current knowledge about the ECG. In 1918 an American physician, James B. Herrick, showed that an abnormal tracing and physical symptoms could indicate a **myocardial infarction** (MI), also known as a heart attack.

Advancements in technology have brought us to today's modern ECG machines. Computer interpretation of the ECG tracing is common. Currently there are ECG machines as small as a wristwatch. Modern ECG machines are easy to use and can provide much information about the heart. An ECG is a common and vital diagnostic tool used worldwide.

Role of an Electrocardiographer

Electrocardiography is an expanding career field. Many health care professionals are trained to record or monitor the heart's electrical activity. These include nurses, physicians, medical assistants, specially trained nursing assistants, and emergency medical personnel. With the changing health care field, other health care employees such as respiratory or radiology personnel are also learning to perform ECGs to improve health care delivery in a variety of health care settings.

Health care personnel who are proficient at recording an ECG can expect to increase their employability and advance their careers. In addition, there are career opportunities for individuals who may want to specialize in the field of electrocardiography. These include, but are not limited to, the ECG technician, the ECG monitoring technician, and the cardiovascular technologist.

An **electrocardiograph (ECG) technician** is an individual who records the ECG and prepares the report for the physician. ECG technicians should be able to determine if the tracing is accurate and recognize abnormalities caused by interference during the recording procedure. Most ECG technicians are employed in hospitals. They may also work in medical offices, cardiac rehabilitation centers, and other health care facilities. In some large hospitals, the ECG technician works in the home health care branch. He or she takes the ECG machine to the patient's home, records the ECG, and gives the report to the physician for interpretation. With the development of multiple tests to evaluate the heart, the ECG technician who obtains continuing education can expect a rewarding career.

Figure 1-2: An ECG monitor technician may be responsible for monitoring multiple patient ECG tracings.

ECG monitor technicians view and evaluate the electrical tracings of patients' hearts on an oscilloscope (see Figure 1-2). ECG monitor technicians are employed at hospitals or other in-patient facilities where patients are attached to continuous or **telemetry** monitors. The main responsibility of an ECG monitor technician is to view the ECG tracings and, if an abnormal heart rhythm occurs, alert the nurse or physician. ECG monitor technicians are required to understand the various heart rhythms and recognize abnormal ones. ECG monitor technicians must be able to evaluate the ECG tracing. They may also be asked to perform other duties such as maintaining patient records and recording ECGs.

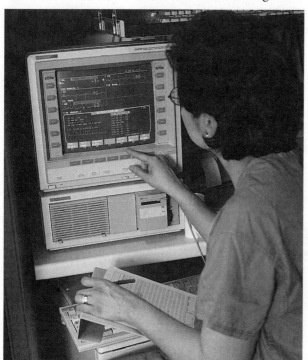

If you enjoy the field of electrocardiology and want to advance your skills or education, you may choose to be a cardiovascular **technologist.** Technologists require more extensive training than technicians. They may assist physicians with invasive cardiovascular diagnostic tests such as **angioplasty,** heart surgery, or implantation of artificial **pacemakers.** Another specialization for cardiovascular technologists is performing ultrasounds on the blood vessels. Ultrasound equipment transmits sound waves, and then collects the echoes to form an image on a screen. As part of their duties, cardiovascular technologists may also perform ECGs.

How ECGs Are Used

Physicians study the ECG tracing to determine many things about the patient's heart. They look for changes from the normal ECG tracing or from the first ECG tracing, which provides a baseline for comparison of subsequent ECGs performed. The American Heart Association recommends that individuals over the age of 40 have an ECG done annually as part of a complete physical. This baseline tracing assists the physician in diagnosing abnormalities of the heart. A sample of a normal tracing is shown in Figure 1-3. We will discuss normal and abnormal ECG tracings in Chapters 2 and 5 of this text.

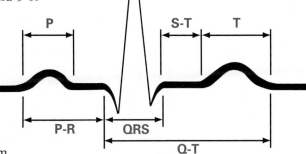

The ECG tracing is recorded using a variety of ECG machines and can be performed in a number of health care settings. These include acute care settings such as hospitals, ambulatory care settings such as clinics or doctor's offices, and even outside of a health care facility. Emergency personnel routinely perform ECGs during emergencies. An ECG tracing can also be transmitted over the telephone from a person's home. The type of ECG tracing produced depends upon the setting and the type of ECG machine used to record.

Figure 1-3: A normal ECG tracing is a straight line with upward and downward spikes or deflections, that indicate electrical activity within the heart.

In the hospital (acute care)

A 12-lead ECG is one of the most common uses of the ECG in the hospital setting. A 12-lead ECG provides a tracing of the electrical activity in the patient's heart at the exact time the ECG tracing is done. In the hospital, a 12-lead ECG is done as a routine procedure or during an emergency such as a **Code Blue.** An emergency ECG may be referred to as "stat," meaning immediately. These are done when a patient experiences chest pain or has a change in his or her cardiac rhythm. Routine ECGs are usually obtained in the early morning so they are available for the physician to review when he or she does morning rounds. Routine ECGs are also frequently done before surgery. Both routine or stat ECGs must be performed safely and with accuracy. The tracing you record will provide critical information about the patient. An inaccurate tracing could result in misdiagnosis, incorrect medications being administered, or other serious outcomes.

Another use of the ECG tracing in the hospital is in continuous monitoring. The purpose of continuous monitoring is to check the pattern of the electrical activity of the patient's heart over time. During continuous monitoring, electrodes are attached to the patient's chest and the tracing is viewed on an oscilloscope. Patients on continuous monitoring are usually in an intensive care unit (ICU), coronary care unit or cardiac care unit (CCU), surgical intensive care unit (SICU), or even an emergency room (ER). Some continuous monitors can also monitor the vital signs and the oxygen level in the blood. Continuous monitoring is also done routinely during surgery.

Another type of continuous monitoring done in a hospital is known as telemetry monitoring. Telemetry monitors are small boxes with electrodes and lead wires

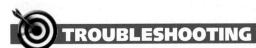

TROUBLESHOOTING

It is essential that you remain calm when recording a "stat" ECG. Remaining calm is necessary to avoid stress to the patient and reduce confusion during the emergency.

attached to the chest. The monitor is usually housed in a case and is attached to the patient so he or she can move about. The ECG tracing is transmitted to a central location for evaluation. When several patients are on a telemetry unit, the tracings of all the patients are recorded on multiple oscilloscopes at the nursing or patient care station.

Performing ECGs in doctors' offices and ambulatory care clinics

A 12-lead ECG is a routine diagnostic test performed in almost any doctor's office or ambulatory care facility. It may be performed as part of a general or routine examination. This routine ECG provides a baseline tracing to be used for comparison if problems arise with a patient. The physician or trained expert looks for changes in a tracing that may indicate different types of health problems. Table 1-2 provides a complete list of conditions that may be diagnosed by an ECG. The procedure for performing a 12-lead ECG is discussed in Chapter 4.

Two other ECG-type tests which may be performed in an office include treadmill stress testing and the ambulatory monitor (**Holter monitor**) (see Figures 1-4 and 1-5).

The treadmill stress test, also known as exercise electrocardiography, is done to determine if the heart gets adequate blood flow during stress or exercise. While the stress test is being performed, the patient is attached to an ECG monitor as he or she is walking on the treadmill. The speed of the treadmill can be varied to measure how this might "stress" the heart. The ECG tracing is recorded and analyzed for changes during the exercise. A physician should always be present during this procedure. The stress test is frequently ordered because it is a safe, noninvasive, inexpensive, and reliable method of measuring the heart's condition if a problem is suspected by the physician. We will discuss the stress test in more detail in Chapter 6.

A Holter monitor is a small box that is strapped to a patient's waist or shoulder to monitor the heart for 24 to 48 hours during a patient's normal daily activity. After the monitoring period, the patient returns to the office for the monitor to be removed. The ambulatory monitor is usually a small tape recorder; however, newer ones on the market are digital. When the recording is finished, it is examined with a special instrument called a scanner. The ECG tracing is then analyzed and interpreted by the physician. We will discuss the ambulatory monitor in detail in Chapter 7.

Outside of a health care facility

Outside of a health care facility, the ECG is a valuable tool used during a cardiac emergency such as a myocardial infarction. Emergency care personnel are equipped with portable ECG machines that can produce an ECG tracing at the

---

Table 1-2 Conditions evaluated by the ECG

- Disorders in heart rate or rhythm and the conduction system
- Presence of electrolyte imbalance
- Condition of the heart prior to defibrillation
- Damage assessment during and after a myocardial infarction (heart attack)
- Disorders of the structure of the heart or coronary blood flow
- Symptoms related to cardiovascular disorders such as weakness, chest pain, or shortness of breath
- Diagnosis of certain drug toxicity
- Diagnosis of metabolic disorders such as hyper- or hypokalemia, hyper- or hypocalcemia, hyper- or hypothyroidism, acidosis, and alkalosis
- Heart condition prior to surgery for individuals at risk for undiagnosed or asymptomatic heart disease
- Damage assessment following blunt or penetrating chest trauma or changes after trauma or injury to the brain or spinal cord
- Assessment of the effects of cardiotoxic or antiarrhythmic therapy
- Suspicion of congenital heart disease
- Pacemaker function

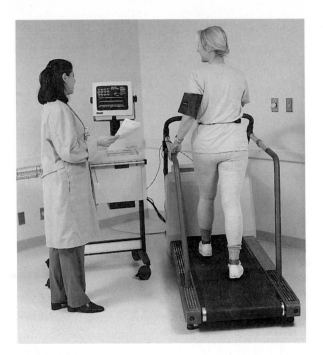

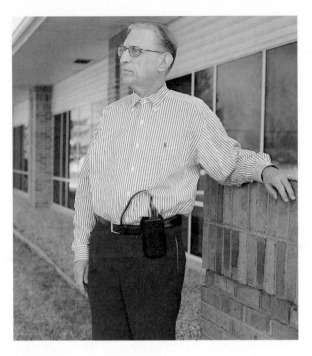

Figure 1-4: This patient is performing a treadmill stress test, also known as exercise electrocardiography. During the exercise, the patient's heart, blood pressure, and oxygen use are being monitored.

Figure 1-5: The Holter or ambulatory monitor allows the patient to participate in routine daily activities while the electrical activity of the heart is being recorded.

site of the emergency. Whether the patient is at home, in a car, or in a crowded football stadium, emergency personnel can monitor and trace the electrical activity of the heart. Figure 1-6 shows one example of a portable ECG machine. In an emergency setting, the tracing can be evaluated for an abnormal ECG pattern. It is either transmitted back to the physician for evaluation or assessed by the emergency medical personnel at the scene. If an abnormal pattern requires immediate treatment, cardiac medications are administered or a **defibrillator** is used. A defibrillator produces an electrical shock to the heart that is intended to correct the heart's electrical pattern. A defibrillator is also commonly used in Code Blue emergencies in the hospital or other health care facilities or site of emergency by appropriate personnel.

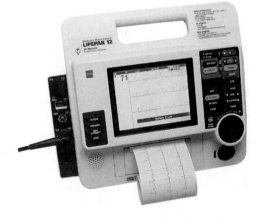

Newer defibrillators can detect abnormal heart rhythms and indicate to the operator when to deliver an electrical shock. These are known as automatic external defibrillators (AEDs) (see Figure 1-7). Many worksites and even airplanes are now equipped with these newer defibrillators. AEDs are easy to use and can quickly provide defibrillation to individuals in any environment. Prior to the availability of AEDs, only specially trained health care professionals could defibrillate the heart. These new machines now make it possible for laypersons to perform defibrillation safely. When the AED's electrodes are placed on the patient's chest, the machine automatically determines the heart rhythm and indicates the need for defibrillation. AEDs produce an electrical shock necessary to correct the heart rhythm. Semiautomatic AEDs require the operator to press a button to perform the actual defibrillation. The use of an AED can increase the heart attack victim's chance for survival.

Another use of the ECG tracing outside of a health care facility is transtelephonic monitoring. Transtelephonic means transmitted (*trans*) over the telephone (*telephonic*). This type of monitoring evaluates the ECG tracing of a patient over time.

Figure 1-6: This portable ECG monitor is transported to the scene during a cardiac emergency and is attached to the patient. The ECG tracing is recorded and viewed by the emergency personnel. In addition, the tracing can be transmitted to the hospital, where a physician can evaluate and determine the necessary drugs and treatment for the patient based upon the heart rhythm viewed.

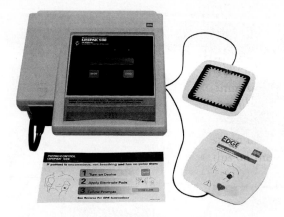

Figure 1-7: Automatic external defibrillators (AEDs) can reverse an abnormal heart rhythm and increase the survival rate of myocardial infarction victims. They can be found in public places and require minimal training to operate.

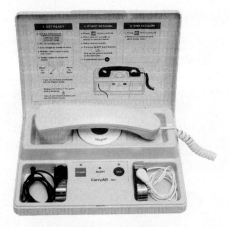

Figure 1-8: Transtelephonic monitors are connected to a telephone at a remote location and the ECG tracing is transmitted and viewed at a central location for interpretation.

Transtelephonic monitoring is useful for patients with symptoms of heart disease that do not occur while they are in the health care facility. These monitors are used for up to 30 days. The small monitors are placed on a telephone mouthpiece and the ECG is transmitted to a health care facility on specific days throughout the monitoring (see Figure 1-8). Individuals using a transtelephonic monitor must understand when and how to record and send a transmission. If your facility provides transtelephonic monitoring, you may be required to teach the patient how to use the monitor. Become familiar with the type of monitor used at your facility.

There are two specific types of transtelephonic monitors. One monitors the heart continuously, and the other records the ECG tracing when the patient is having symptoms. Continuous transtelephonic monitoring is programmed to record the ECG tracing constantly. It is useful to record the ECG tracing before, during, and after a patient has symptoms. These symptoms may include chest pain, shortness of breath, dizziness, or palpitations. This type of monitor is a small device that attaches to the patient's chest with two electrodes. The smallest monitor available is about the size and shape of a beeper.

Symptom-based transtelephonic monitoring is in the form of either a handheld or a wristwatch device. The handheld type has electrode feet that are pressed against the patient's chest after symptoms occur. Currently one type is as small as a credit card and can be carried in a pocket or wallet. The wristwatch type monitor is worn on the left arm at all times. The patient must turn on this type of monitor when symptoms begin.

Transtelephonic monitoring is generally used to evaluate artificial pacemaker functioning. In addition, monitors are sometimes given to patients after an emergency room visit. If the patient has symptoms of cardiac problems but is not admitted to the hospital, a physician will often give the patient a monitor to record an ECG when the symptoms recur. It is less expensive to give patients a monitor to take home than to admit them to the hospital.

What You Need to Know to Perform an ECG

In order to perform an ECG you should become familiar with the procedure and the ECG machine. You must have the ability to lift and move the patient, if necessary. You need to be able to transport and operate the ECG machine. In addition, you must understand basic principles of safety and infection control, patient education and communication, and law and ethics. Being able to troubleshoot problems or situations that arise during the procedure is also essential.

Equipment

Knowing how to use the equipment is part of performing an ECG. You must be able to transport, operate, maintain, and store the ECG equipment used at your facility. There are many different machines available to perform an ECG, and directions provided by the manufacturer are an important source of information. Many ECG machines have reference cards or instructions posted in a convenient place on or with the equipment. Refer to these printed materials when performing an ECG. Although all ECG machines are similar, you should become familiar with the particular machine you are using. You should always perform at least one or two practice ECGs before using any machine on a patient. Since an ECG is noninvasive, you can practice on a volunteer, friend, co-worker, or fellow student.

Safety and infection control

When performing health care procedures, you must always maintain the safety of yourself and the patient. General safety guidelines should be followed at all times. Certain safety precautions specific to performing the ECG procedure should also be followed. These specific precautions will be discussed in more detail in Chapter 4.

SAFETY AND INFECTION CONTROL - Follow safety and infection control guidelines at all times when working in a health care facility and performing an ECG.

Universal Precautions

Preventing the spread of infection is an essential part of providing health care and performing an ECG. This is for your safety as well as for the safety of your patients. Guidelines to prevent the spread of infection are called *Universal Precautions.* Properly performed Universal Precautions can prevent the transfer of infection from one patient to another, from the common cold to more serious infections such as **hepatitis** or **HIV.** Universal Precautions are based on recommendations made by the Centers for Disease Control and Prevention (CDC) and are mandated by the Occupational Safety and Health Administration (OSHA) to lower the risk of occupational disease transmission. OSHA is the federal agency responsible for ensuring that all employees work in safe environments. The CDC studies infectious diseases and determines the necessary precautions to prevent disease transmission. Universal Precautions are practiced in all employment situations in which exposure to blood or body fluids is likely. Universal Precautions are used for all patients with or without an identified infection. Table 1-3 (on pg. 10) provides a list of Universal Precautions that should be practiced when recording an ECG.

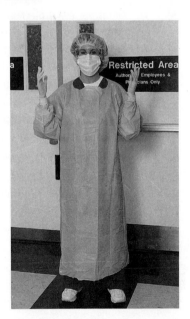

Standard Precautions

At an in-patient facility such as a hospital, Standard Precautions are practiced on patients with known or suspected infections. Standard Precautions, which include rules for isolated patients, are the combination of Universal Precautions and Body Substance Isolation. Body Substance Isolation, recommended by the CDC, is designed to reduce the risk of transmission of pathogens from moist body substances. Standard Precautions apply to (1) blood; (2) all body fluids, secretions, and excretions except sweat, regardless of whether or not they contain visible blood; (3) nonintact skin; and (4) mucous membranes. Standard Precautions include the use of barrier devices, called personal protection equipment, when caring for patients in isolation. These include gloves, gown, mask, and eye protection (see Figure 1-9).

As a health care provider, you must always follow Universal Precautions regardless of where you work. Standard Precautions include rules that apply to isolated patients in hospitals with known or suspected infections. Specific information about Standard Precautions related to recording an ECG will be included in Chapter 4.

Figure 1-9: Personal protection equipment (PPE) is used to reduce the risk of transmission of infection. PPE includes items such as gloves, mask, gown, and eye protection.

Table 1-3 Universal Precautions related to electrocardiography

Hand Washing

- Wash your hands after touching blood, body fluids, secretions, excretions, and contaminated items.
- Wash your hands before putting on gloves and after removing gloves.
- Wash your hands between patient contacts.
- Wash your hands between tasks and procedures on the same person.

Gloves

- Wear gloves when touching blood, body fluids, secretions, excretions, and contaminated items.
- Wear gloves when touching mucous membranes and nonintact skin.
- Change gloves between procedures and patients.
- Change gloves after contacting materials that are highly contaminated.
- Remove gloves promptly after use.
- Remove gloves before touching uncontaminated surfaces or items.
- Wash your hands immediately after glove removal.

Masks, Eye Protection, and Face Shields

- Masks, eye protection, and face shields protect the mucous membranes of the mouth, eyes, and nose from splashes and sprays.
- Wear mask, eye protection, and face shields during procedures and tasks that are likely to cause splashes or sprays of blood, body fluids, secretions, and excretions.

Gowns

- Gowns protect the skin and clothing.
- Wear a gown during procedures and activities that are likely to cause splashes or sprays of blood, body fluids, secretions, or excretions.
- Remove a soiled gown promptly.
- Wash your hands immediately after gown removal.

Equipment

- Equipment may be soiled with blood, body fluids, secretions, and excretions.
- Handle used equipment carefully.
- Prevent skin and mucous membrane exposure and clothing contamination.
- Reusable equipment must be cleaned, disinfected, or sterilized before it is used on another person.
- Discard single-use equipment promptly.

Environmental Control

- Follow facility procedures for the routine care, cleaning, and disinfection of surfaces. This includes environmental surfaces, nonmovable equipment, and other frequently touched surfaces.

Occupational Health and Bloodborne Pathogens

- Use resuscitation devices for mouth-to-mouth resuscitation.

Patient education and communication

Communicating with your patients is key to successfully recording an ECG. You must develop a positive relationship and atmosphere to reduce apprehension and anxiety during an ECG. You can reduce the patient's fears and make the ECG a positive experience by developing a helpful relationship with your patients and practicing effective communication techniques. Clearly explaining the procedure and answering questions are essential for good patient communication. Maintain a friendly, confident manner while interacting with your patient. Your patient will be more cooperative if he or she trusts you are competent to perform your job.

Helping the patient understand the procedure and follow instructions is essential to performing any ECG procedure. When explaining the procedure, use simple terms and speak slowly and distinctly. Encourage the patient to ask questions and repeat the instructions. This process will help ensure patient understanding.

In addition, in your role as a multiskilled health care professional, you will need to be able to work in a variety of situations, as a team member, and be able to resolve conflicts. As with any job, you should continue to improve in your performance through further education and practice.

SAFETY AND INFECTION CONTROL - Hand washing is the single most important procedure you can perform to prevent the spread of infection. When practicing Universal Precautions and wearing gloves, you must wash your hands before putting gloves on and after removing them to prevent disease transmission.

Legal and ethical issues

As a multiskilled health care professional, you must understand some legal and ethical considerations of patient care. Laws are rules of conduct that are enforced by a controlling authority such as the government. An unlawful act can result in loss of your job, a fine, or other penalty such as time in jail. Ethics are concerned with standards of behavior and concepts of right and wrong. They are based upon moral values that are formed through the influence of the family, culture, and society. Unethical acts result in poor job evaluations or job loss. When comparing law and ethics you should understand that illegal acts are always unethical, but unethical acts are not always illegal.

Practicing ethics

Many professions have a code of ethics. These are standards of behavior or conduct as defined by the professional group. As a health care professional, you must follow the standards of behavior or code of ethics set forth by your profession and place of employment. The following are some basic ethics you should practice.

Confidentiality is an essential part of patient care. You may collect information about a patient for use during his or her care and treatment; however, this information should not be made public. Confidentiality is a basic right of every patient. You should not speak about your patients or allow information about your patients to be heard or seen by anyone other than those caring for them. A breach in confidentiality is both unethical and illegal.

Patients should be treated with respect and dignity. You should respect the privacy of patients at all times. Avoid exposing your patient's body when performing any procedure by closing the door, pulling the curtain, and/or draping the patient.

Practicing ethics also includes professionalism, respect, and cooperation. You should maintain professionalism by continuing your education and training in order to provide the highest level of care for your patient. You should respect your patient's beliefs, values, and morals, and work cooperatively with your co-workers and supervisors at all times.

Legal issues you should know

Medical professional liability means that a health care professional is legally responsible for his or her performance. Health care professionals can be held accountable for performing unlawful acts, performing legal acts improperly, or simply failing to perform an act when they should. For example, if you find a patient's wallet after he or she leaves and you decide to keep it, this is an illegal act. While you are assisting with a treadmill stress test, if you report the blood pressure results incorrectly, resulting in the patient having a severe heart attack, this is performing a legal act improperly. If you decide to take a break when you are supposed to be monitoring a patient's heart rhythm and during the time you are gone the patient experiences an abnormal heart rhythm resulting in death from lack of prompt treatment, you have failed to perform your duties as required.

You will be speaking and writing about patients as part of your job as an electrocardiographer. You should never speak defamatory words about patients even when they upset you. Making derogatory remarks about a patient—or anyone else—that jeopardizes his or her reputation or means of livelihood is called slander. Slander is an illegal and unethical act that could cause you to lose your job. If you write defamatory words, this is known as libel, which is also illegal and unethical.

PATIENT EDUCATION AND COMMUNICATION - When speaking to a patient who is hard of hearing, look directly at the patient and speak slowly and distinctly. The patient may be able to read your lips. When your patient speaks another language, you may want to ask an interpreter or family member to assist you with communication thus reducing apprehension and anxiety.

LAW AND ETHICS - The patient's chart should not be left out or open in an area where other patients or visitors may be able to view it. This is a breach of confidentiality.

Table 1-4 Required entries for medical records related to ECG

- Patient identification, including full name, social security number, birth date, full address and telephone number, marital status, and place of employment, if applicable
- Patient's medical history
- Dates and times of all appointments, admissions, discharge, and diagnostic tests such as an ECG
- Diagnostic test results
- Information regarding symptoms and reason for appointment, diagnostic test, or admission
- Physician examinations and record of results, including patient instructions
- Medications and prescriptions given, including refills
- Documentation of informed consent when required
- Legal guardian or representative, if patient is unable to give informed consent

Medical care and treatment must be documented as part of the medical record. The medical record can be used in court as evidence in a medical professional liability case. To protect yourself legally and provide continuity of patient care, you should include complete information in the medical record. See Table 1-4 for a complete list of the necessary information to document on the medical record.

Whatever ECG procedure you are performing, the patient must agree or consent to having the procedure done. Implied consent is between the patient and health care professional such as a physician in an office. For example, when a patient requests care and comes to the physician's office, he or she is agreeing to be treated by the physician. This is *implied* consent. When a patient agrees to the ECG procedure, this is also implied consent.

Certain diagnostic procedures, including a treadmill stress test, require *informed* consent. The patient must understand the procedure and its associated risks, alternative procedures and their risks, and the potential risks to the patient if he or she refuses treatment. Informed consent requires the patient to sign a consent form.

Troubleshooting

When caring for patients and recording an ECG you may experience a variety of problems. These problems may stem from the patient's condition, patient communication, equipment failure, or other complications. While performing an ECG, you may need to troubleshoot actual or potential complications during the procedure. Troubleshooting requires critical thinking. Critical thinking is the process of thinking through the situation or problem and making a decision to solve it. Let us say that you are about to perform an ECG and the patient refuses to let you attach the lead wires. As part of troubleshooting, you ask the patient why he or she is refusing. The patient states, "I do not want that electricity going through me!" In a calm manner, you explain that the machine does not produce or generate electricity and it is not harmful. After your explanation, the patient agrees to have the ECG. You have performed successful troubleshooting. Throughout this text, various situations will be discussed and potential solutions given. In each chapter review the "What Would You Do?" questions to check your ability to think critically and troubleshoot.

⊙ TROUBLESHOOTING

When a patient who cannot read or write is required to sign a consent form, you will need to explain the procedure to a family member and have that person sign and the patient sign unless he or she has been determined to be incompetent. If this is not possible, explain the procedure to the patient with a witness present and have the witness sign, along with having the patient place an X on the form.

Chapter Review

The Match Game: Match these terms with the correct definition. Place the appropriate letter on the line to the left of each term.

_____ 1. cardiovascular

_____ 2. electrocardiogram

_____ 3. arrhythmia

_____ 4. electrocardiology

_____ 5. electrocardiograph

_____ 6. defibrillator

a. An instrument used to record the electrical activity of the heart.

b. A tracing of the signal produced by the heart's electrical activity and used for diagnostic evaluation of the heart.

c. The study of the heart's electrical activity.

d. Abnormal or absence of normal heartbeat, also known as dysrhythmia.

e. Related to the heart and blood vessels (veins and arteries).

f. A machine that produces and sends an electrical shock to the heart that is intended to correct the electrical pattern of the heart.

Make Them True: Read each statement and determine if it is true or false. Place a T or F on the line provided. For each of the false (F) statements, correct them to "make them true."

_____ 7. An ECG machine produces and records the electrical activity of the heart.

_____ 8. Standard Precautions are guidelines written for health care providers to help prevent the spread of infection.

_____ 9. When performing an ECG you should know the equipment, infection control principles, communication techniques, and safety guidelines.

_____ 10. A transtelephonic monitor transmits an ECG over the Internet.

It's Your Choice: Circle the correct answer.

11. The first ECG machine was developed in _____ by _____. He won the Nobel Prize for this invention.

    a. 1903, Wilhelm Einthoven

    b. 1918, James B. Herrick

    c. 1876, Augusta D. Waller

    d. 1945, Sir Thomas Lewis

12. Which of the following is *not* a reason for performing an ECG?

    a. to evaluate heart conditions

    b. to check for problems with the flow of electricity through the heart

    c. to see how well the heart is contracting and pumping

    d. to evaluate the rate and rhythm of breathing

13. A continuous monitor is used most commonly in a:

    a. physician's office

    b. hospital

    c. assisted-living center

    d. clinic

14. Which of the following is most commonly performed in a clinic or hospital?

    a. transtelephonic monitor

    b. ambulatory monitor

    c. 12-lead ECG

    d. defibrillator

15. To write derogatory words about a patient is known as:

    a. slander

    b. libel

    c. ethical

    d. unethical

16. Your most important duties include recording an ECG and preparing the report for the physician. You are most likely a(n):

    a. ECG monitor technician

    b. cardiovascular technologist

    c. ECG technician or medical assistant

    d. physician's assistant

What Would You Do?

Read the following situations and use critical thinking skills to determine how you would handle each. Write your answer in detail in the space provided.

17. You have been performing ECGs at a local clinic for about 6 months. Your favorite uncle says to you, "Since I just turned 40, your Aunt Beth thinks I should have an ECG. Will you do one on me if I come by where you work?" What would you say or do for your uncle? Consider the following:

    Should your uncle have an ECG? _____

    Should you do the ECG if he stops by your office? Why or why not? _____

    _____

    _____

    _____

18. Mr. Smith has been having some mild chest pain. During his ECG, he says, "How does it look? Is there anything wrong?" What would be your best response?

    _____

    _____

    _____

19. You walk by a room where a co-worker is performing an ECG on a female patient. The door is open and the patient is not covered. What would you do?

_____

_____

_____

20. You are responsible for monitoring the heart rhythms on six patients at a local hospital when you begin to feel ill. You are in desperate need to go to the restroom and you really want to go home. What should you do?

_____

_____

_____

_____

GET CONNECTED TO THE WEB

History of the ECG If you would like to learn more about the history of the ECG, check out this site:
- ECG Library: A brief history of electrocardiography (http://homepages.enterprise.net/djenkins/ecghist.html)

Career Exploration If you would like to obtain more information about a career as cardiovascular technologist or technician, visit the Bureau of Labor Statistics Occupations Outlook Handbook at this site:
- http://stats.bls.gov/oco/ocos100.htm

Automatic Defibrillators To learn more about automatic external defibrillators, visit the American Heart Association's site at http://www.americanheart.org and search for the keyword *AED* or *automatic external defibrillator.*

Risk Factors Go to the http://www.americanheart.org site and click on the heart and stroke A–Z guide, and then click on biostatistical fact sheets. Identify at least 5 cardiovascular facts related to a specific cultural group and/or identify 5 risk factors for cardiovascular disease and what can be done to reduce the risk of disease for each. (If you would like to know about the American Heart Association located in your state, add the state's initials at the end of the Internet site; for example, http://www.americanheart.org/va/.)

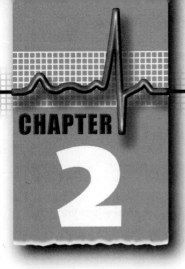

CHAPTER 2

The Cardiovascular System

Objectives

Upon completion of this chapter, you should be able to:

▶ Identify the structures of the heart including valves, chambers, and vessels

▶ Compare and contrast the pulmonary and systemic circulation

▶ Trace the pathway of the blood through pulmonary and systemic circulation

▶ Describe coronary circulation

▶ Explain the cardiac cycle

▶ Identify what takes place during systole and diastole

▶ Describe the parts and function of the conduction system

▶ Define the unique qualities of the heart and their relationship to the cardiac conduction system

▶ Explain the conduction system as it relates to the ECG

▶ Discuss the electrical stimulation of the heart as it relates to the ECG waveform

▶ Identify each part of the ECG waveform

▶ Describe the heart activity that produces the ECG waveform

Key Terms

aorta - The largest artery of the body, which transports blood from the left ventricle of the heart to the entire body.

aortic semilunar valve - Valve located in the aorta that prevents the backflow of blood into the left ventricle.

atrioventricular (AV) node - Specialized cells that delay the electrical conduction through the heart and allow the atria time to contract.

atrium (pl. atria) - One of the upper two small chambers of the heart. The right atrium receives blood from the body through the vena cava, and the left atrium receives blood from the lungs through the pulmonary vein.

automaticity - The ability of the heart to initiate an electrical impulse without being stimulated by another source.

bundle branches - Left and right branches of the Bundle of His that conduct impulses down either side of the interventricular septum to the left and right ventricles.

Bundle of His (AV bundle) - A bundle of fibers that originate in the AV node and enter the interventricular septum conducting electrical impulses to the left and right bundle branches.

cardiac cycle - The period from the beginning of one heartbeat to the beginning of the next; the cardiac cycle is made up of systole and diastole.

Key Terms (cont.)

complex - A group of ECG waveform deflections that indicate electrical activity in the heart.

conductivity - The ability of the heart cells to receive and transmit an electrical impulse.

contractility - The ability of the heart muscle cells to shorten in response to an electrical stimulus.

coronary circulation - The circulation of blood to and from the heart muscle.

deoxygenated blood - Blood that has little or no oxygen (oxygen-poor blood).

depolarization - The electrical activation of the cells of the heart that initiates contraction of the heart muscle.

diastole - The phase of the cardiac cycle when the heart is expanding and refilling; also known as the relaxation phase.

excitability - The ability of the heart muscle cells to respond to an impulse or stimulus.

interval - The period of time between two activities within the heart.

interventricular septum - A partition or wall (septum) that divides the right and left ventricles.

ischemia - Temporary lack of blood supply to an area of tissue due to a blockage in the circulation to that area.

isoelectric - The period when the electrical tracing of the ECG is at zero or a straight line; no positive or negative deflections are seen.

left atrium - The left upper chamber of the heart, which receives blood from the lungs.

left ventricle - The left lower chamber of the heart, which pumps oxygenated blood through the body; also known as the workhorse of the heart.

mitral (bicuspid) valve - Valve with two cusps or leaflets located between the left atrium and left ventricle; it prevents backflow of blood into the left atrium.

myocardial - Pertaining to the heart (*cardi*) muscle (*myo*).

oxygenated blood - Blood having oxygen (oxygen-rich blood).

pericardium - A two-layered sac of tissue enclosing the heart.

polarization - The state of cellular rest in which the inside is negatively charged and the outside is positively charged.

pulmonary artery - Large artery that transports deoxygenated blood from the right ventricle to the lungs; the only artery in the body that carries deoxygenated blood.

pulmonary circulation - The transportation of blood to and from the lungs; blood is oxygenated in the lungs during pulmonary circulation.

pulmonary semilunar valve - A valve found in the pulmonary artery that prevents backflow of blood into the right ventricle during pulmonary circulation.

pulmonary vein - A blood vessel that transports blood from the lungs to the left atrium. The only vein in the body to carry oxygenated blood.

Purkinje fibers - The fibers within the heart that distribute electrical impulses to cells throughout the ventricles.

Purkinje network - A network of fibers that distribute electrical impulses through the ventricles; named after a scientist with the last name of Purkinje.

repolarization - When heart muscle cells return to their resting electrical state and the heart muscle relaxes.

right atrium - The right upper chamber of the heart, which receives blood from the body.

right ventricle - The right lower chamber of the heart, which pumps blood to the lungs.

segment - A portion or part of the electrical tracing produced by the heart.

semilunar valve - A valve with half-moon-shaped cusps that open and close, allowing blood to travel only one way; located in the pulmonary artery and the aorta.

sinoatrial (SA) node - An area of specialized cells in the upper right atrium that initiates the heartbeat.

systemic circulation - The circulation between the heart and the entire body excluding the lungs.

systole - The contraction phase of the cardiac cycle, during which the heart is pumping blood out to the body.

tricuspid valve - Valve located between the right atrium and right ventricle; it prevents backflow of blood into the right atrium.

vena cava - Largest vein in the body, which provides a pathway for deoxygenated blood to return to the heart; its upper portion, the superior vena cava, transports blood from the head, arms, and upper body; and its lower portion, the inferior vena cava, transports blood from the lower body and legs.

The function of the heart is to pump blood to and from all the tissues of the body. Blood supplies the tissues with nutrients and oxygen and removes carbon dioxide and waste products. The process of transporting blood to and from the body tissues is known as circulation. The heart's powerful muscular pump performs the task of circulation. Circulation of the blood is dependent upon the heart and its ability to contract or beat. Each contraction of the heart is recorded on the ECG. Knowledge of the heart, its functions, and what produces the ECG tracing will provide you with a clear understanding of the tasks you will be performing as an ECG health care professional.

Anatomy of the Heart

The heart lies in the center of the chest, under the sternum, and in between the lungs. Two-thirds of it lies to the left of the sternum. It is approximately the size of your fist and weighs about 10.6 ounces or 300 grams (see Figure 2-1).

The heart is a powerful muscular pump that beats an average of 72 times per minute, 100,000 times per day, and 22.5 billion times in the average lifetime. The heart pumps about 140 mL of blood per beat, for a total output of 5 liters per minute. Each day the heart pumps approximately 7250 liters or 1800 gallons of blood. This is enough to fill an average size bathtub about 36 times.

The entire heart is enclosed in a sac of tissue called the **pericardium.** This sac consists of two layers: the tough, outer layer is called the parietal layer and the inner layer is called the visceral layer. The visceral pericardium adheres closely to the heart. It is also referred to as the epicardium, the outermost layer of the heart. The purpose of the pericardium is to protect the heart from infection and trauma. The space between the two layers is called the pericardial space. It contains about 10–20 mL (about 1/2 ounce) of fluid. This fluid serves to cushion the heart against blows and decreases friction between the layers created by the pumping heart.

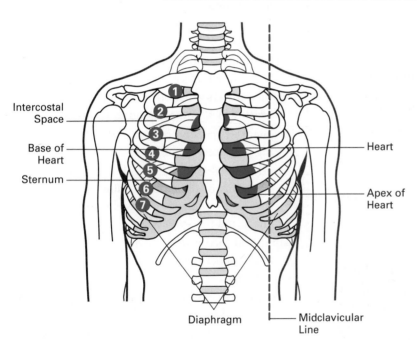

Intercostal Space

Base of Heart

Sternum

Heart

Apex of Heart

Diaphragm

Midclavicular Line

Figure 2-1: The heart is tipped to the left side of the body, and two-thirds of it is located on the left side of the chest.

The heart consists of three layers: the endocardium, the myocardium, and the epicardium or visceral pericardium. The epicardium, the outermost layer, is thin and contains the coronary arteries. The myocardium is the middle muscular layer that contracts the heart. The endocardium is the innermost layer, which lines the inner surfaces of the heart chambers and the valves. It is also where the Purkinje fibers are located (see Figure 2-2 and Table 2-1).

Chambers and valves

The heart is divided into four chambers. The top chambers are the **right atrium** and **left atrium.** The bottom chambers are the **right ventricle** and **left ventricle.** The myocardium varies in thickness between chambers. It is thin in the atria, thick in the

Table 2-1 **Heart layers**	
Layer	**Location and Function**
Endocardium	Inner layer of the heart that lines the chambers and valves. The Purkinje fibers are located here.
Myocardium	Middle, thickest muscular layer, responsible for heart contraction
Epicardium (also called the visceral pericardium)	Outside, thin layer of the heart that contains the coronary arteries; also the inner layer of the pericardium
Pericardium (made up of the visceral pericardium and the parietal pericardium)	A double-layer sac that encloses the heart. The inner layer, or visceral pericardium, is also called the epicardium; the outer layer is the parietal pericardium.

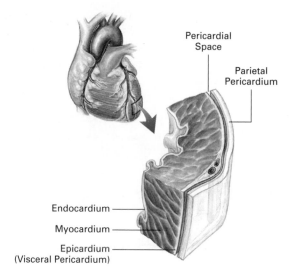

Figure 2-2: Three distinct layers can be identified on the heart. A sac called the pericardium protects it.

right ventricle, and thickest in the left ventricle. The thicker the myocardium of a chamber is, the stronger the muscular contraction of that chamber. The left ventricle is sometimes known as the "workhorse of the heart" because of its thick myocardium and powerful muscular contraction.

Between the right atrium and right ventricle is the **tricuspid valve.** Between the left atrium and left ventricle is the **mitral (bicuspid) valve.** These two valves are known as atrioventricular valves because they divide the atria from the ventricles. The **pulmonary artery** and the **aorta** each have a **semilunar valve.** They are called semilunar because the valve flaps look like a half (*semi*) moon (*lunar*). These valves are called the **aortic semilunar valve** and the **pulmonary semilunar valve** (see Figure 2-3 and Table 2-2).

The one-way valves in the heart keep the blood flow headed in the right direction. The flaps or "cusps" open to allow the blood to flow, then close to prevent the back-flow of blood. The mitral (bicuspid) and tricuspid valves separate the atria and ventricles and prevent the blood from flowing back from the ventricles to the atria.

Table 2-2 **Heart valves and their locations**		
Name	**Valve Type**	**Location**
Aortic	Semilunar	Between left ventricle and aorta
Pulmonary	Semilunar	Between right ventricle and pulmonary artery
Tricuspid	Atrioventricular	Separates right atrium and right ventricle
Mitral (bicuspid)	Atrioventricular	Separates left atrium and left ventricle

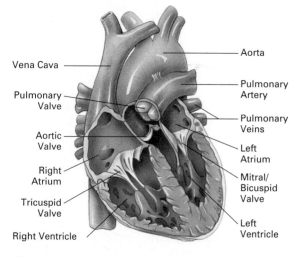

Figure 2-3: Heart chambers, valves, and vessels

The Cardiovascular System | 19

The semilunar valves in the pulmonary artery and the aorta prevent the backflow of blood into the ventricles (see Figure 2-4).

The major vessels of the heart

Blood vessels are the veins and arteries that transport blood all over the body. The major blood vessels that transport blood to and from the heart are the vena cava, pulmonary artery, pulmonary veins, and the aorta.

Blood travels from the body tissue through the veins toward the heart. The blood is returned through the largest vein of the body, the **vena cava,** to the right atrium. There are two branches to the vena cava. The superior vena cava transports blood from the head, arms, and upper body. The inferior vena cava transports blood from the lower body and legs.

When the heart contracts, the right ventricle pumps **deoxygenated blood** (blood that has little or no oxygen) to the lungs via the pulmonary artery. The **pulmonary veins** transport **oxygenated blood** (blood containing oxygen) back to the heart into the left atrium. Transporting blood to the entire body is the function of the aorta. When the left ventricle contracts, the blood is pumped into the aorta. The first vessels to branch off the aorta are the coronary arteries. Coronary arteries are part of coronary circulation, which supplies blood to the muscular heart pump (see Figure 2-5).

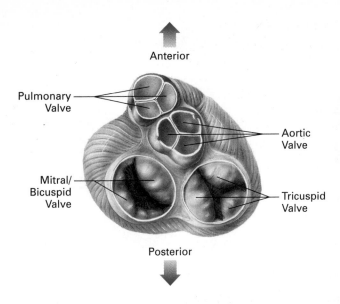

Figure 2-4: Valves viewed from a cross section of the heart

Principles of Circulation

The heart is actually a two-sided pump. The left side of the heart pumps oxygenated blood to the body tissue. The right side of the heart pumps deoxygenated blood to the lungs. The pathways for pumping blood to and from the lungs are known as **pulmonary circulation.** The pathways for pumping blood throughout the body and back to the heart are known as **systemic circulation.** The circulation of blood to and from the heart muscle is known as **coronary circulation.**

Pulmonary circulation: The heart and lung connection

Deoxygenated blood enters the right atrium through the superior and inferior vena cava. Blood travels through the tricuspid valve into the right ventricle. The right ventricle pumps the blood through the pulmonary semilunar valve into the pulmonary artery, then into the lungs. In the lungs, the blood is oxygenated. The blood returns to the heart through the pulmonary veins into the left atrium. The left atrium is the last step of pulmonary circulation.

Systemic circulation: The heart and body connection

Oxygenated blood enters the left atrium and travels through the mitral valve into the left

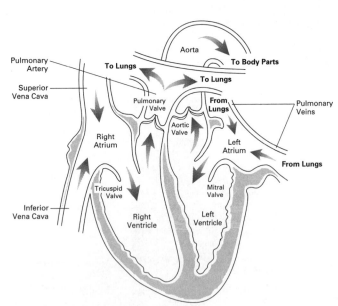

Figure 2-5: Pathways for blood through the heart

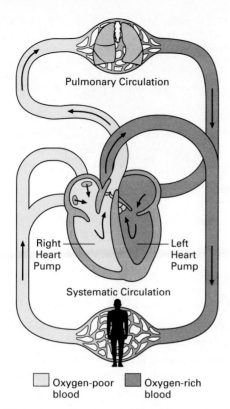

Pulmonary Circulation

Right Heart Pump

Left Heart Pump

Systematic Circulation

☐ Oxygen-poor blood   ■ Oxygen-rich blood

Figure 2-6: Pulmonary and systemic circulation

ventricle. The left ventricle pumps the blood through the aortic semilunar valve into the aorta. The aorta provides the pathway for the blood to circulate through the body. In the body, the oxygen in the blood is exchanged with carbon dioxide. After traveling through the body, the deoxygenated blood returns to the heart through the superior and inferior vena cava (see Figure 2-6).

Coronary circulation: The heart's blood supply

Oxygenated blood from the left ventricle travels through the aorta to the coronary arteries. There are two main coronary arteries, the left main artery and the right main coronary artery. These arteries branch to supply oxygenated blood to the entire heart. The left main artery has more branches than the right because the left side of the heart is more muscular and requires more blood supply. The deoxygenated blood travels through the coronary veins and is collected in the coronary sinus, which empties the blood directly into the right atrium (see Figure 2-7).

The Cardiac Cycle

Each beat of the heart has two phases that indicate the contraction and the relaxation periods of the heart. The contraction and relaxation of the heart together make up the **cardiac cycle.** When the heart contracts, it is squeezing blood out to the body. As the heart relaxes, it is expanding and refilling. The relaxation phase of the heart is known as **diastole.** The contraction phase is known as **systole** (see Figure 2-8 on p. 22).

Diastole: Relaxation of the heart

During the diastolic phase, blood from the upper body returns to the heart via the superior vena cava and blood from the lower body returns via the inferior vena cava. The right atrium fills with blood and contracts, pushing open the tricuspid valve. This allows blood to flow into the right ventricle. At the same time, blood is returning from the lungs via the pulmonary veins to the left atrium. This blood fills the left atrium prior to the atrial contraction. The atrial contraction forces the mitral valve open to allow blood to flow into the left ventricle.

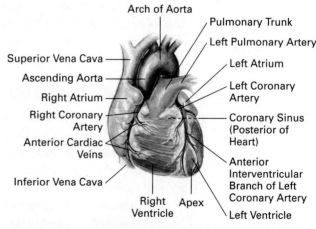

Figure 2-7: Coronary circulation

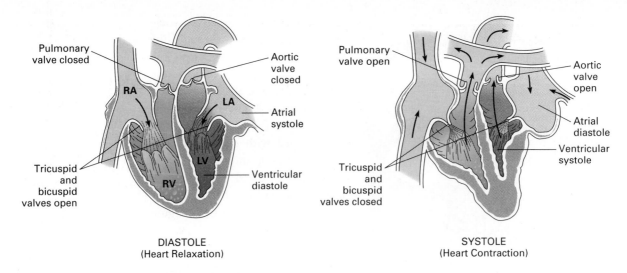

Pulmonary
valve closed

Aortic
valve
closed

RA

LA

Atrial
systole

Tricuspid
and
bicuspid
valves open

LV

RV

Ventricular
diastole

DIASTOLE
(Heart Relaxation)

Pulmonary
valve open

Aortic
valve
open

Atrial
diastole

Tricuspid
and
bicuspid
valves closed

Ventricular
systole

SYSTOLE
(Heart Contraction)

Figure 2-8: Diastole and systole

Systole: Contraction of the heart

During the systolic phase, the heart muscle contracts, creating pressure to open the pulmonary and aortic valves. Blood from the right ventricle is pushed into the lungs to exchange oxygen and carbon dioxide. Blood from the left ventricle is pushed through the aorta to be distributed throughout the body to provide oxygen for tissues and remove carbon dioxide.

In adults, the average heart beats approximately 60 to100 times per minute. In general, women have a faster heartbeat than men. Children's heart rates are usually faster than an adult's heart rate. Children's heart rates depend upon the age and size of the child. If you listen to the heart with a stethoscope, you will hear two sounds: "lubb" and "dupp." These sounds are made by the opening and closing of the heart valves, which is caused by the contraction of the heart. The "lubb" you hear is the sound made during the systolic phase by the contraction of the ventricles and the closing of the mitral and tricuspid valves. The "dupp" sound is made during the diastolic phase. It is shorter and occurs during the beginning of ventricular relaxation. This sound is from the closure of the pulmonary and aortic valves. Each complete "lubb-dupp" you hear is actually one beat of the heart.

Conduction System of the Heart

The pumping cycle or contraction of the heart muscle is controlled by electrical impulses. These impulses are initiated and transmitted through the heart. Specialized masses of tissue in the heart produce these impulses and form the conduction system. The conduction system is necessary for the heart to pump continuously and rhythmically.

Unique qualities of the heart

The conduction system is a network of conducting tissue that creates the heartbeat and establishes a pattern for the electrical activity of the heart. The conducting tissue of the heart has several unique qualities. These qualities control the beat of the heart and produce the electrical wave. They include automaticity, conductivity, contractility, and excitability.

Automaticity is the ability of the heart to initiate an electrical impulse without being stimulated by another or independent source. Automaticity is a form of the word *automatic,* which is exactly how the heart beats—automatically. The heart tissue has its own innate ability to initiate an electrical impulse.

The heartbeat relies on the ability of the **myocardial** cells to conduct electrical impulses. (**Myocardial** means pertaining to the heart muscle.) **Conductivity** is the ability of the heart cells to receive and transmit an electrical impulse. The electrical impulse is initiated by automaticity and then travels through the rest of the heart due to the ability of the heart cells to conduct the impulse.

When the heart muscle cells are stimulated by an electrical impulse, they contract. This ability of the heart muscle cells to shorten in response to an electrical stimulus is known as **contractility.** The contraction of the heart muscle cells produces the heartbeat or pumping of the heart.

Excitability is the ability of the heart muscle cells to respond to an impulse or stimulus. Without the quality of excitability, the heart would not react to the electrical impulses that are initiated within the heart.

As you can see, the heart's unique qualities are essential to the rhythmic contraction of the heart muscle and the circulation of blood through the body. Without these qualities the heart would not beat.

In addition to automaticity, the heartbeat is controlled by the autonomic nervous system (ANS). Like the unique qualities of the heart, the ANS is involuntary. This means you have no conscious control over its functions. The sympathetic branch of the ANS increases the heart rate. This happens automatically when you are under stress or become frightened. You can think of the automaticity of the heart as the cruise control in your car. In a normal heart, automaticity sets the rate of the heart to 60 to 100 beats a minute. When the sympathetic branch of the ANS is stimulated, it speeds up the heart. When you let your foot off the accelerator (remove the stimulation to the sympathetic branch of the ANS), the heart rate coasts down to the cruise control speed of 60 to 100.

The parasympathetic branch of the ANS exerts a depressant effect on the heart. The vagus nerve is the major nerve of the parasympathetic system and exerts an effect on many of the body organs. It is widespread throughout the body. Stimulation of the vagus nerve slows the heart, acting like a brake to the heart rate. When a patient is experiencing an abnormally fast heart rate, stimulation of the vagus nerve is used to bring the heart back to its normal cruise control rate.

Pathways for conduction

The conduction system consists of the sinoatrial (SA) node, atrioventricular (AV) node, Bundle of His (AV bundle), bundle branches, and the Purkinje fibers (network). The SA and AV nodes are small, round structures that consist of Purkinje fibers. The **sinoatrial (SA) node** is located in the upper portion of the right atrium. It is the pacemaker of the heart and initiates the heartbeat. The automaticity of the fibers in the SA node produces the contraction of the right and left atria. The SA node fires at about 60 to 100 times per minute. Normal conduction of the heart begins with the SA node (see Figure 2-9 and Table 2-3 on p. 24).

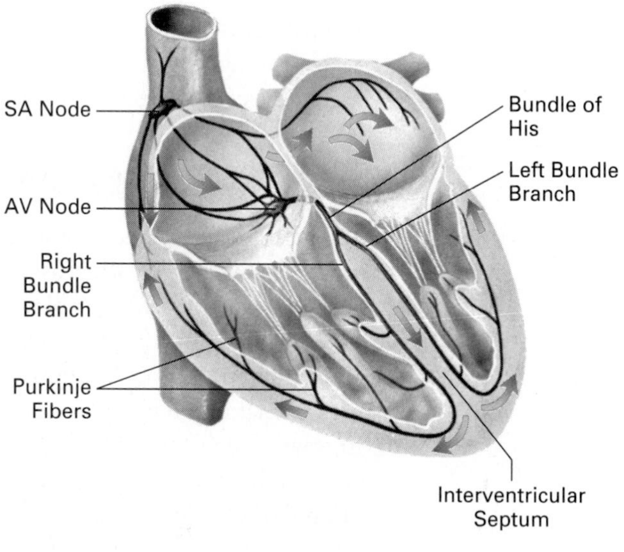

On the floor of the right atrium is another mass of Purkinje fibers known as the **atrioventricular (AV) node.** Impulses travel to the AV node because of the unique quality of conductivity through a specialized

Figure 2-9: Conduction pathways

SA Node

AV Node

Right Bundle Branch

Purkinje Fibers

Bundle of His

Left Bundle Branch

Interventricular Septum

Table 2-3 Parts of the conduction system

Part	Function
Sinoatrial (SA) node (pacemaker)	Initiates heart at a rate of 60 to100 beats per minute with electrical impulse that causes depolarization
Atrioventricular (AV) node	Delays the electrical impulse to allow for the atria to complete their contraction and ventricles to fill before the next contraction
Bundle of His (AV bundle)	Conducts electrical impulses from the atria to the ventricles
Bundle branches	Conducts impulses down both sides of the interventricular septum
Purkinje fibers (network)	Distributes the electrical impulses through the right and left ventricles

pathway through the atria. The AV node itself causes a delay (slowdown) in the electrical impulse. This process is important for two reasons. First, it provides time for additional blood to travel from the atria to the ventricles before they contract. This additional blood is known as the atrial kick. The atrial kick increases the cardiac output or the amount of blood that is pumped out of the heart into the body with each contraction. Second, the delay in the electrical impulse reduces the number of electrical impulses transmitted to the ventricles. This is important when the atria is firing too fast. It prevents an excessive rate of electrical impulses from reaching the ventricles. The AV node can also act as the pacemaker if the SA node is not working. It will fire at a rate of 40 to 60 times per minute. This is known as the inherent rate of the AV node.

The **Bundle of His (AV bundle),** located next to the AV node, provides the transfer of the electrical impulse from the atria to the ventricles. When the impulse reaches the ventricles, it is divided into the bundle branches. The **bundle branches** are located along the left and right side of the **interventricular septum.** The electrical impulse travels through the right and left bundle branches to the right and left ventricles. The bundle branches are like a fork in the road, and the electrical impulse splits and travels down both sides.

The right and left bundle branches are pathways down the interventricular septum, where the impulses travel to activate the myocardial tissue to contract. Impulses traveling down the left bundle branch will stimulate the interventricular septum to contract in a left-to-right pattern. The ventricles receive their electrical impulses from the bundle branches.

The **Purkinje network** spreads the impulse throughout the ventricles, which occurs through a network of fibers called the **Purkinje fibers.** These fibers provide an electrical pathway for each of the cardiac cells. The electrical impulses accelerate and activate the right and left ventricles at the same time to cause the ventricles to contract. The electrical impulse produces an electrical wave.

Electrical Stimulation and the ECG Waveform

Heart cells, in their resting state, are electrically polarized. This means their insides are negatively charged, whereas on the outside, they are positively charged. This state of cellular rest is known as **polarization** and is the ready phase of the heart.

Depolarization, on the other hand, is a state of cellular stimulation, which precedes contraction. It is the electrical activation of the cells of the heart when they lose their internal negativity. Depolarization moves from cell to cell through the electrical pathways. Depolarization is the most important electrical event in the heart—it causes the heart to contract and pump blood to the body.

Repolarization is a state of cellular recovery, which follows each contraction. The cardiac cells return to their resting phase of internal negativity. After depolarization, the cardiac cells return to this state in order to prepare for another depolarization. During repolarization the heart relaxes and allows for refilling of the chambers of the heart.

The ECG waveform is recorded from the electrical activity produced during depolarization and repolarization of the heart. The waveform on the electrocardiogram is a series of up-and-down deflections off a straight line known as an **isoelectric** line. The isoelectric line represents the period when no electrical activity is occurring in the heart and is known as a baseline. Deflections, which appear as waves on the ECG tracing, indicate electrical activity in the heart. The deflections that go up are positive; the deflections that go down are negative.

When the waveform was first discovered, Einthoven labeled the waves of the electrocardiogram as P, Q, R, S, and T. Legend holds that he chose the letters from the center of the alphabet because he did not know what the waves meant, or whether other waves preceding the P wave or following the T wave would be discovered. The U wave was added after Einthoven's discovery. Each of these waves indicates specific activity in the heart (see Table 2-4).

In addition to the waves, the ECG waveform contains **intervals, segments,** and **complexes.** Each of these elements indicates specific activity within the heart. The elements include the QRS complex, the ST segment, the PR interval, and the QT interval.

What each part of the waveform represents

The first deflection is positive and is known as the P wave. This P wave is seen when the atria depolarize. The P wave is small (compared to the other waves of the ECG), rounded, and is the first wave of the normal complex.

During the delay of conduction that occurs at the AV node, a small baseline segment is seen on the waveform. There is no electrical activity occurring (depolarization or repolarization), thus no wave or deflection is seen. It is during this time that atrial kick occurs.

The Q wave represents the conduction of the impulse down the interventricular septum. It is a negative deflection before the R wave. It is not unusual or abnormal for a QRS complex not to have a Q wave. A normal Q wave is less than one fourth

Table 2-4 **ECG components**		
Component	**Appearance**	**Heart Activity**
P wave	Upward small curve	Atrial depolarization with resulting atrial contraction
QRS complex	Q, R, and S waves	Ventricular depolarization and resulting ventricular contraction (larger than the P wave) atrial repolarization occurs (not seen)
T wave	Small upward sloping curve	Ventricular repolarization
U wave	Small upward curve	Repolarization of the Bundle of His and Purkinje fibers (not always seen)
PR interval	P wave and baseline prior to QRS complex	Beginning of atrial depolarization to the beginning of ventricular depolarization; time it takes the impulse to travel from the SA node to the AV node
QT interval	QRS complex, ST segment, and T wave	Period of time from the start of ventricular depolarization to the end of ventricular repolarization
ST segment	End of QRS complex to the beginning of T wave	Time between ventricular depolarization and the beginning of ventricular repolarization

of the height of the R wave. The R wave is the first positive wave. It represents the conduction of electrical impulse to the left ventricle. It is usually the easiest wave to locate on the ECG tracing. The S wave is the first negative deflection after the R wave. It represents the conduction of the electrical impulse through both ventricles. The QRS waves together form the QRS complex. The QRS complex represents ventricular depolarization. It is reflective of the time it takes for the impulses to activate the myocardium to complete contraction from the Purkinje fibers.

The ST segment is measured from the end of the S wave to the beginning of the T wave. This segment should normally be on the isoelectric line. It indicates the end of ventricular depolarization and the beginning of ventricular repolarization. The reason this segment is studied in a 12-lead ECG recording is to determine whether or not there is any ischemia and myocardial damage. **Ischemia,** which is a lack of oxygen to the heart muscle, causes the ST segment to elevate. An elevated ST segment indicates myocardial damage in the form of injury to the heart muscle. These changes are studied when interpreting an ECG. More information about interpreting an ECG is included in Chapter 5.

The T wave represents ventricular repolarization. As repolarization occurs, the ventricular muscles relax. Normal T waves are in the same direction as the QRS complex and the P wave. A normal T wave peaks toward the end instead of the middle. Unlike the symmetrical mountain shape of the P wave, the T wave looks like a small mountain with one sloping side.

The U wave follows the T wave. The U wave represents repolarization of the Bundle of His and Purkinje fibers. The U wave does not always show up on the ECG; however, its presence can indicate an electrolyte imbalance.

The PR interval is measured from the beginning of the P wave to the beginning of the QRS complex. The normal length of time for the PR interval is 0.12 to 0.20 seconds. The PR interval on a normal ECG should be consistent.

The QT interval is the time required for ventricular depolarization and repolarization to take place. It begins at the beginning of the QRS complex and ends at the end of the T wave. It includes the QRS complex, ST segment, and the T wave.

R to R interval is the measurement of time from the start of a QRS complex in a rhythm to the start of the next adjacent QRS complex. R waves are readily seen on the ECG and are used to calculate the heart rate in a regular rhythm. We will discuss this in Chapter 3.

The junction of the QRS interval and the ST interval is the J point. This represents the end of the QRS complex and ventricular depolarization. The J point is important when measuring the length of the QRS complex and interpreting the ECG tracing. A normal QRS complex is .06 to .10 seconds (see Figure 2-10).

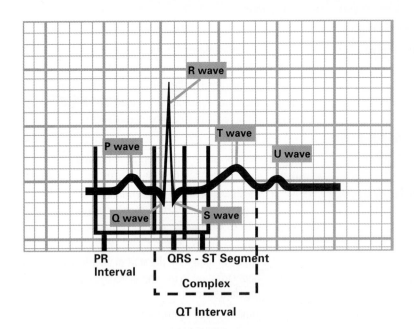

Figure 2-10: The ECG waveform and heart activity

Chapter Review

The Match Game: Match the valves, vessels, and chambers of the heart to their definitions. Place the correct letter on the line provided.

_____ 1. left ventricle

_____ 2. tricuspid valve

_____ 3. left atrium

_____ 4. aorta

_____ 5. pulmonary artery

_____ 6. right atrium

_____ 7. right ventricle

_____ 8. semilunar valve

_____ 9. pulmonary vein

_____ 10. mitral valve

a. artery that transports blood to the entire body

b. type of valve located in the aorta and the pulmonary artery

c. atrioventricular valve between the left atrium and left ventricle

d. heart chamber that pumps blood to the body, known as the workhorse of the heart

e. heart chamber that receives blood from the lungs

f. chamber of the heart that receives blood from the body

g. chamber of the heart that pumps blood to the lungs

h. blood vessels that transport blood from the lungs to the left atrium

i. valve located between the right atrium and right ventricle

j. blood vessel that provides a pathway for deoxygenated blood to return to the lungs

Match the conduction system parts and unique qualities of the heart to their definitions. Place the correct letter on the line provided.

_____ 11. excitability

_____ 12. automaticity

_____ 13. bundle branches

_____ 14. SA node

_____ 15. contractility

_____ 16. depolarization

_____ 17. AV node

_____ 18. Purkinje fibers

_____ 19. repolarization

_____ 20. conductivity

a. delays the electrical conduction through the heart

b. ability of the heart to initiate an electrical impulse

c. branches off the Bundle of His that conduct impulses to the left and right ventricle

d. ability of the heart cells to receive and transmit an electrical impulse

e. an electrical current that initiates the contraction of the heart muscle

f. ability of the heart muscle cells to shorten in response to an electrical stimulus

g. ability of the heart muscle cells to respond to an impulse or stimulus

h. heart muscle cells return to their resting electrical state and the heart muscle relaxes

i. initiates the heartbeat

j. distributes electrical impulses from cell to cell throughout the ventricles

21. The PR interval is usually:

    a. .06 to .10 seconds

    b. .12 to .20 seconds

    c. greater than .20 seconds

    d. less than .06 seconds

22. What part of the ECG tracing represents the repolarization of the Bundle of His and Purkinje fibers?

    a. T wave

    b. PR interval

    c. U wave

    d. P wave

23. What part of the ECG tracing represents the time it takes for the impulse to activate the myocardium to the complete contraction?

    a. QRS complex

    b. J point

    c. QT interval

    d. PR interval

24. What part of the ECG tracing is measured from the end of the S wave to the beginning of the T wave and is normally on the isoelectric line?

    a. ST segment

    b. QT segment

    c. U wave

    d. QRS complex

25. What wave on the ECG tracing is not always seen and sometimes when seen can indicate an electrolyte imbalance?

    a. U wave

    b. P wave

    c. Q wave

    d. R wave

The Match Game Part Two: Match the information about circulation and the cardiac cycle to the definitions. Place the correct letter on the line provided.

_____ 26. deoxygenated blood

_____ 27. cardiac cycle

_____ 28. systole

_____ 29. coronary circulation

_____ 30. systemic circulation

_____ 31. oxygenated blood

_____ 32. diastole

_____ 33. pulmonary circulation

a. period between the beginning of one beat of the heart to the next

b. circulation of blood through the heart and heart muscle

c. blood that has little or no oxygen

d. phase of the cardiac cycle when the heart is expanding and refilling; also known as the relaxation phase

e. blood having oxygen

f. circulation between the heart and the entire body, excluding the lungs

g. transportation of blood to and from the lungs

h. contraction phase of the cardiac cycle, when the heart is pumping blood out to the body

Label the Parts

34. a.–l. Label the vessels, valves, and chambers of the heart by using the letters of the terms.

a. Right atrium

b. Aorta

c. Right ventricle

d. Pulmonary veins

e. Left atrium

f. Left ventricle

g. Vena cava

h. Pulmonary valve

i. Aortic valve

j. Tricuspid valve

k. Pulmonary artery

l. Mitral (bicuspid valve)

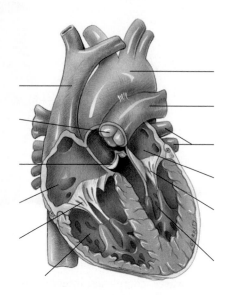

35. Label the following figure representing the flow of blood through the heart. Use the letters of the terms.

a. Superior vena cava

b. Right atrium

c. Aorta

d. Right ventricle

e. Pulmonary valve

f. Left atrium

g. Lungs

h. Mitral valve

i. Pulmonary vein

j. Tricuspid valve

k. Left ventricle

l. Aortic valve

m. Pulmonary artery

n. Inferior vena cava

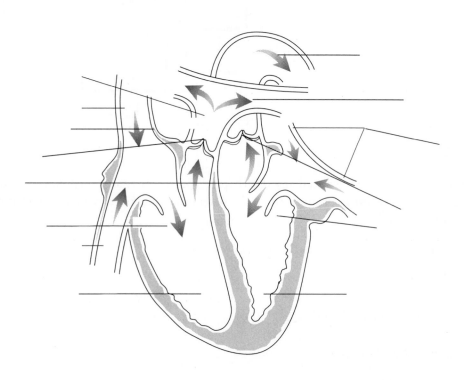

36. a.–g. Label the parts of the conduction system.

a. Inteventricular septum
b. Left bundle branch
c. Purkinje fibers
d. AV node
e. SA node
f. Bundle of His
g. Right bundle branch

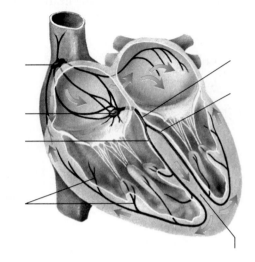

37. a.–j. Label the waves, complexes, intervals, and segments of the ECG waveform.

a. S wave
b. R wave
c. P wave
d. U wave
e. T wave
f. Q wave
g. QT interval
h. Complex
i. QRS-ST interval
j. PR interval

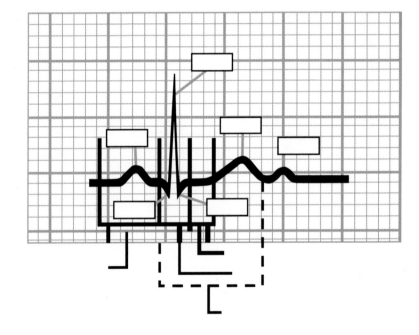

Right or Wrong?

38. You and a friend have just finished studying this chapter. Your friend makes the following statements. Are his or her statements correct or incorrect? If the statement is incorrect, write down what you would say to correct your friend.

a. "The valves between the atria and the ventricles are semilunar." _____

_____

b. "The atria always pump the blood." _____

_____

c. "The heart is a two-sided pump that produces pulmonary circulation and systemic circulation."

_____

d. "The coronary arteries carry deoxygenated blood."_____

_____

e. "The pulmonary artery carries oxygenated blood."_____

_____

f. "The waves on the ECG waveform are positive when they are up and negative when they are down."

_____

g. "If you are a man you will have a faster heartbeat."_____

_____

h. "The top chambers of the heart are the ventricles and the bottom chambers of the heart are the atria."_____

_____

i. "The right ventricle is sometimes known as the workhorse of the heart."_____

_____

j. "The waves of the ECG waveform are P, Q, R, S, T, and sometimes a U."_____

_____

Voyage Through the Heart

39. For each of the following statements, identify the vessel or structure you are in. Write in the space provided. Imagine you are a drop of blood traveling through the heart. Returning from the brain, you are about ready to enter the heart.

a. What vessel are you in?_____

_____

b. After you enter the right atrium, you have to go through a door in order to enter the right ventricle. What is the name of this door?_____

_____

c. You have made it to the lungs successfully and are traveling back to the heart. What vessels are you in?_____

_____

d. When you get to the heart where will you be? _____

_____

e. You have finally made it to the last chamber of the heart. The left ventricle pumps you into the entire body. After entering the aorta, what are the very first vessels you will travel into?

_____

_____

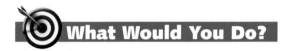

What Would You Do?

Read the following situations and use your critical thinking skills to determine how you would handle each. Write your answer in detail in the space provided.

40. When the atria outside of the SA node stimulates the atria to beat too fast, this is known as atrial flutter or atrial fibrillation. When these heart rhythms occur, the ventricles do not beat at the same rate as the atria. What part of the conduction system prevents the ventricles from beating as fast as the atria and how does it occur?

_____

_____

41. You are working in the emergency room recording an ECG when the electricity goes out. There is a short period of darkness followed by a very loud noise. When you regain power, the heart of you and your patient are beating extremely fast. What part of the cardiovascular system is responsible for this increased heart rate? Should you continue recording the ECG now or later, and why?

_____

_____

GET CONNECTED TO THE WEB

Learn More About the Heart For more information about the heart and some real-life pictures, go to the Web site Heart: A Virtual Exploration at http://sln.fi.edu/biosci/heart.html.

The site Heart Info, at http://www.heartinfo.org/physician/ecg/norm.htm, shows a normal 12-lead ECG and the parts of the ECG waveform along with what they represent. Go to this site to review the ECG waveform.

At the University of Utah's site http://medstat.med.utah.edu/ WebPath/CVHTML/CVIDX.html you can view pictures of the heart and its structures. Go to this site and find the pictures of the heart valves. Describe each valve, where it is located, and how it functions.

Search the National Heart, Lung, and Blood Institute's Web site at http://www. nhlbi.nih.gov/ for more information about coronary heart disease.

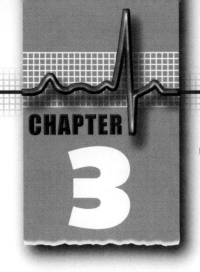

CHAPTER 3

The Electrocardiograph

Objectives

Upon completion of this chapter, you should be able to:

▶ Identify the three types of leads

▶ Explain how each lead is recorded

▶ Compare and contrast the differences between a single channel and a multichannel ECG machine

▶ List the functions of common ECG machines

▶ Discuss the ECG machine controls and identify how each control is used

▶ Describe the parts of the electrocardiograph

▶ Identify common electrodes and electrolyte products

▶ Describe the ECG graph paper

▶ Identify the measurements of an ECG waveform on the ECG graph paper

Key Terms

artifact - Unwanted marks on the ECG tracing caused by activity other than the heart's electrical activity.

augmented - Normally small ECG lead tracings that are increased in size by the ECG machine in order to be interpreted.

bipolar - A type of ECG lead that measures the flow of electrical current in two directions at the same time.

bradycardia - A slow heart rate, usually less than 60 beats per minute.

Einthoven triangle - A triangle formed by three of the limb electrodes—the left arm, the right arm, and the left leg; it is used to determine the first six leads of the 12-lead ECG.

electrodes - Small sensors, metal plates, or disposable units placed on the skin during an ECG to receive the electrical activity from the heart.

gain - A control on the ECG machine that increases or decreases the size of the ECG tracing.

input - Data entered into an ECG machine, usually through electrodes on the surface of the skin.

lead - A conductor attached to the ECG machine in the form of a covered wire.

limb - An arm or a leg.

mm (millimeter) - A unit of measurement to indicate time on the ECG tracing. Time is measured on the horizontal axis.

multichannel recorder - An ECG machine that has the ability to record more than one lead tracing at a time, usually 3, 4, or 6.

mV (millivolt) - A unit of measurement to indicate voltage on the ECG tracing. Voltage is measured on the vertical axis.

Key Terms (cont.)

oscilloscope - A TV or monitor type device that shows the tracing of the electrical activity of the heart.

output display - The part of the ECG machine that displays the tracing for the electrical activity of the heart, usually in a printed form on a 12-lead ECG machine.

precordial - A type of lead placed on the chest in front of the heart; known as a V lead.

signal processing - The process within the ECG machine that amplifies the electrical impulse and converts it to a mechanical action on the output display.

single-channel recorder - An ECG machine that records one lead tracing at a time.

speed - A control on the ECG machine to regulate how fast or slow the paper runs during a tracing.

standardization - Setting of the ECG machine output so that 1 millivolt equals 1 centimeter.

stylus - A pointed, penlike instrument that uses heat to record electrical impulses on the ECG graph paper.

tachycardia - A fast heart rate, usually greater than 100 beats per minute.

unipolar - A type of ECG lead that measures the flow of electrical current in one direction only.

In Chapter 2 you learned about the heart's conduction system and how the ECG waveform is produced. In this chapter we will discuss the electrocardiograph and the equipment needed to perform an ECG and record the ECG waveform. You will discover how the 12-lead system works and what the measurements are on the ECG graph paper. Learning the equipment and lead system thoroughly and correctly will prepare you to record your first ECG.

Producing the ECG Waveform

The electrical impulse that is produced by the heart's conduction system is measured with the ECG machine. The ECG machine interprets the impulse and produces the ECG waveform. The waveform indicates how the heart is functioning. Since the heart is three dimensional, it is necessary to view the electrical impulse and heart functioning from different sides. A single heart rhythm views the heart from one angle. A 12-lead ECG is a complete picture of the heart's electrical activity, looking at it from 12 different angles as you might look at a sculpture. It records the heart's electrical activity in 12 different views at slightly different angles. The 12-lead ECG records the electrical impulses produced in the heart. It is not a picture of the heart structure; it is a recording of the electrical activity within the heart. The 12 views provide information about how the electrical impulses travel through various parts of the heart.

A 12-lead ECG is actually recorded by only 10 lead wires, which, when attached to the chest and the **limbs** (arms and legs), provide the 12 different views for the 12-lead tracing. Six of these leads attach to the chest electrodes, and the other four attach to the electrodes on the arms and legs. **Electrodes** are small sensors placed on the skin to receive the electrical activity from the heart, and **leads** are covered wires that conduct the electrical impulse from the electrodes to the ECG machine. The lead wires are identified by color and are labeled

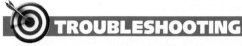

TROUBLESHOOTING

Each of the lead wires is coded by color and letter. If you place the lead wires incorrectly, the ECG will not record at all or it will record the waveforms improperly. Always check and double-check the lead wires before you begin the tracing. An ECG recording produced with the lead wires attached incorrectly is not acceptable and will have to be repeated.

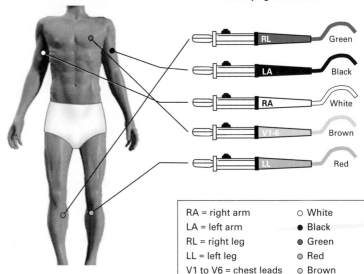

Table 3-1 **Lead identification**		
Identifying Letters	**Designated Color**	**Lead Wire Placement**
RA	White	Right arm
LA	Black	Left arm
RL	Green	Right leg
LL	Red	Left leg
V1-V6	Brown	Chest leads

RA = right arm   ○ White
LA = left arm   ● Black
RL = right leg   ◑ Green
LL = left leg   ◎ Red
V1 to V6 = chest leads   ○ Brown

with letters to match the correct position on the patient's body (see Table 3-1 and Figure 3-1).

The 10 lead wires produce 12 different lead circuits consisting of one or more wires from the electrodes to the electrocardiograph. The 12 circuits produce 12 different tracings or views of the heart. The electrodes, or a combination of electrodes, identify each of the 12 leads. The 12 leads are made up of three different types of leads: three standard limb leads, three augmented leads, and six chest leads.

To understand the circuits for the first six leads (three standard and three augmented) we can use the Einthoven triangle. Einthoven is the scientist credited with developing the first ECG machine. The **Einthoven triangle** is formed by three of the limb electrodes: those on the right arm, the left arm, and the left leg. The right leg is used only as a ground or reference electrode (see Figure 3-2).

The electrical current created by the heart is measured between the positive and negative electrodes placed on the body. If no current is flowing, the waveform is flat, or isoelectric. If the current moves toward the positive electrode, the ECG waveform will be positive, or upright, above the isoelectric baseline. If the current moves away from the positive electrode or toward the negative electrode, the ECG waveform will be negative, or downward, below the isoelectric baseline.

Figure 3-1: When attaching the lead wires, check carefully for the correct color- and letter-coded wire.

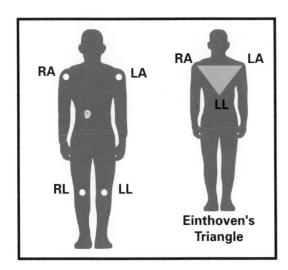

Einthoven's Triangle

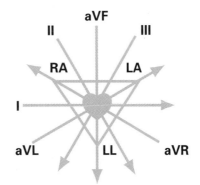

Figure 3-2: The Einthoven triangle helps us understand the reference points for the 12-lead ECG.

Standard limb leads

The first three leads are known as standard limb leads. They are also known as **bipolar** leads because they measure the flow of electrical current in two directions at the same time. These first three leads are called lead I, lead II, and lead III. In the Einthoven triangle, leads I, II, and III are positioned at the same distance from the heart's electrical activity. Lead I records the tracing from the right arm (-) to the left arm (+) and produces a positive wave. Lead II records the tracing from the right arm (-) to the left leg (+) and produces a positive or upward deflection. Lead III records the electrical activity traveling from the left arm (-) to the left leg (+) (see Figure 3-3).

Augmented leads

The second three leads are known as **augmented** leads because their tracings are increased in size by the ECG machine in order to be interpreted. They are also known

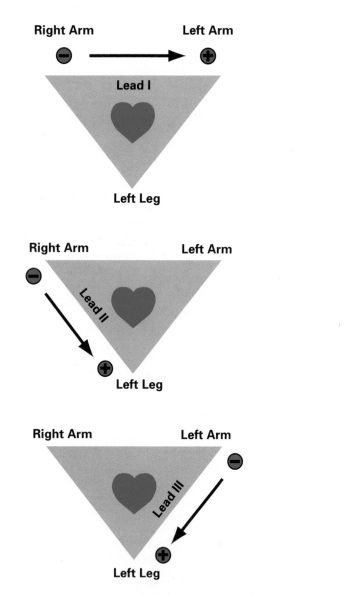

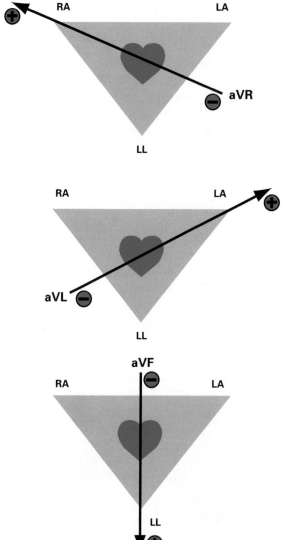

Figure 3-3: Leads I, II, and III are standard limb leads and are recorded from these reference points on the Einthoven triangle.

Figure 3-4: The augmented leads aVR, aVL, and aVF are recorded from midway between two points on the Einthoven triangle. Because of the lead reference points, their tracings are normally small but are augmented (enlarged) by the ECG machine.

as **unipolar** leads because they measure toward one electrode on the body. They are called aVR, aVL, and aVF. The R, L, and F refer to the direction the lead is measuring: R is right arm, L is left arm, and F is foot (see Figure 3-4). Lead aVR records electrical activity from midway between the left arm and left leg to the right arm. Lead aVR is usually a negative deflection. If it does not produce a negative deflection, you might have the electrodes or lead wires placed incorrectly. To ensure accuracy of electrodes and lead wire placement, check the aVR tracing produced when recording the 12-lead ECG; if it is not a negative deflection, change the placement of the electrodes and lead wires to correct it.

Lead aVL records electrical activity from the midpoint between the right arm and left leg to the left arm. Lead aVF records electrical activity from the midpoint between the right arm and left arm to the left leg. The voltage is very low with the augmented leads because of the angle of measurement; therefore the ECG waveform will be very small. The ECG machine must increase (augment) the size of the waveforms for these leads to be readable on the ECG tracing.

Chest leads

The last six leads are the chest leads. Also known as **precordial,** these leads are located in front of (*pre*) the heart (*cor*). The chest leads are unipolar because they are measured in one direction only. They are placed on specific sites on the chest. Each of the chest leads begins with the letter V and is numbered from V1 to V6. These leads record activity between six points on the chest and within the heart. The correct placement of these leads is essential in obtaining an accurate tracing (see Figure 3-5). Exact physical placement of the lead wires and electrodes on the limbs and chest will be discussed in Chapter 4.

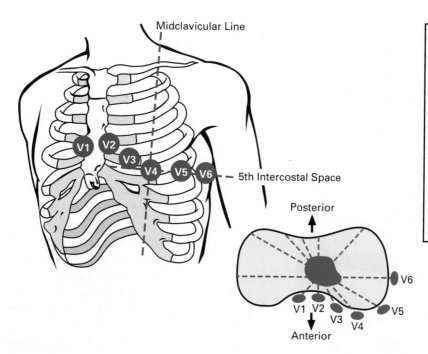

V1 - fourth intercostal space, right sternal border
V2 - fourth intercostal space, left sternal border
V3 - halfway between V2 and V4
V4 - fifth intercostal space at the midclavicular line
V5 - on the same horizontal level with V4, at the anterior axillary line
V6 - on the same horizontal level with V4 and V5, at the midaxillary line

Figure 3-5: Front and cross section view of chest lead placement.

The 12-lead ECG tracings can be interpreted separately or in conjunction with each other. When an ECG is being recorded, each of the 12 leads must be identified on the tracing. Older machines required that the ECG tracing strip be coded with identifying marks manually. Newer machines identify each lead tracing automatically. Each lead tracing looks slightly different and presents a different picture of the heart. This allows the physician to determine damage or problems in specific areas of the heart (see Figure 3-6 on p. 38).

Figure 3-6: A 12-lead ECG produced on a multichannel ECG machine. Each lead is identified on the printout. Note the difference in appearance of the tracings from the 12 leads.

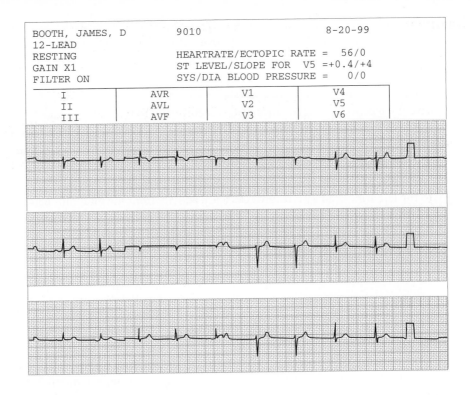

```
BOOTH, JAMES, D        9010                    8-20-99
12-LEAD
RESTING              HEARTRATE/ECTOPIC RATE  =   56/0
GAIN X1              ST LEVEL/SLOPE FOR  V5 =+0.4/+4
FILTER ON           SYS/DIA BLOOD PRESSURE =   0/0
```

I	AVR	V1	V4
II	AVL	V2	V5
III	AVF	V3	V6

ECG Machines

Machines used today to measure an ECG weigh less than 10 pounds; some are as small as a credit card. All ECG machines vary slightly, but most have the same basic parts. The typical ECG machine sits on a small cart that can be pushed to the person requiring the ECG. You should become familiar with the type of machine you will be using by reading the manufacturer's instructions.

Types of ECG machines

Figure 3-7: A single-channel ECG machine records only one lead at a time and uses a roll of paper that produces a single lead strip.

There are two main types of ECG machine recorders: single-channel recorders and multichannel recorders. The **single channel recorder** monitors 12 leads individually; it produces a strip three to six feet long showing all 12 leads (see Figure 3-7). The recorded ECG tracing strip must be cut and mounted, or placed on a card, for interpretation. Each lead is marked on the strip while the ECG is recording. The ECG tracing must be mounted correctly to ensure proper interpretation by the physician. Read the directions carefully and place each lead tracing in the correct location. Mounting a single-channel ECG tracing will be discussed in more detail in Chapter 4.

The **multichannel,** three-channel ECG **recorder** monitors all 12 leads but records three leads at once and switches automatically, recording each of the four sets of three leads. As seen in Figure 3-6, it produces a full sheet of paper showing all 12 lead tracings. The actual recording time for this machine is approximately ten seconds (see Figure 3-8). This tracing does not usually need to be mounted, but it may need to be attached to a thicker backing when filed permanently. Also available are newer multichannel ECG machines that can record up to six lead tracings at one time.

Functions

There are three basic functions of the electrocardiograph: input, signal processing, and output display. Sensors in the ECG machine serve as receiving devices for the electrical activity of the heart. Electrodes placed on the patient's skin direct the impulses to the ECG instrument, providing the **input** for the ECG machine.

Signal processing occurs inside the ECG machine. It amplifies the electrical impulse and converts it into mechanical actions on the display. A complex collection of transistors, resistors, and circuitry amplify and prepare the signal for transfer to the output display.

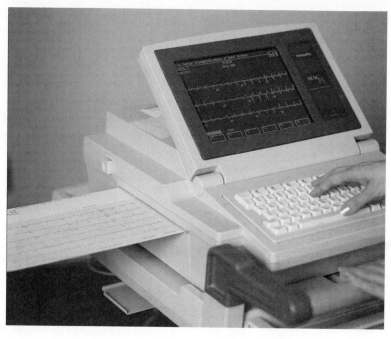

Figure 3-8: A multichannel ECG machine records 3, 4, or 6 leads at a time on a large sheet of ECG graph paper.

The **output display** is the result of the ECG tracing. Most commonly, this is the printed report. In some cases, the output also appears on a screen known as an **oscilloscope.** An oscilloscope is frequently found on a cardiac monitor or a defibrillator. For a 12-lead ECG, the printed format is the most important output display since it provides a hard copy of the information.

Newer ECG machines perform other functions as well, including computerized measurement and analysis, storage, and communication. Computerized measurement and analysis provide a machine interpretation of the ECG. This interpretation is not meant to replace the physician's interpretation. However, the computer interpretation can distinguish between a normal and abnormal recording quickly, and may provide a second opinion.

Some ECG machines store ECG results, which can be recalled and printed later. ECG machines are also equipped to transmit results over the telephone, fax, or Internet. As new technology is being developed, you should stay current on the latest changes and advancements.

Controls

The three most important controls on the electrocardiograph include the speed, gain, and artifact filter.

Speed

The **speed** control regulates how fast or slow the paper runs during the ECG procedure. The most commonly used standard rate is 25 millimeters per second (written as 25 **mm**/sec). In some cases you may want to increase the speed to 50mm/sec,

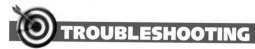
TROUBLESHOOTING

When the patient's heart rate is very fast, it will be difficult to read the ECG tracing because the waveform parts will be close together. Set the speed control at 50 mm/sec to widen the complexes so the ECG can be interpreted more easily. Be sure to note this on the ECG report.

which is twice as fast. You would do this if the patient has an unusually rapid heart rate. It may also be done if the ECG waveform parts are too close together. Increasing the speed would allow the waveform to be analyzed more easily. Some ECG machines allow you to reduce the speed to 5mm/sec or 10mm/sec in order to analyze the ECG recording more carefully. Changing the speed of the recorder would only be done at the request or preference of the physician. Remember, if you change the speed to anything other than the standard 25 mm/sec, you should note this on the tracing.

Gain

The **gain** control regulates the output or height of the ECG waveform. The normal setting is 10mm/**mV** (millivolts are the units of measurement used to indicate voltage on the ECG tracing). By setting the gain to 20mm/mV, you can double the size; by setting the gain to 5mm/mV, you reduce the size by half. Some machines will let you change the gain depending on which lead you are tracing. Since the tracing size can vary between lead, setting the gain will allow the ECG waveform to be readable for any lead tracing. If you change the gain setting during any lead tracing, you must record this change on the ECG report.

Artifact filter

The ECG machine you are using may have an **artifact** filter selection. The usual setting is between 40 Hz (hertz, a unit of frequency) and 150 Hz. Forty Hz is normally used to reduce artifact, or abnormal marks on the ECG tracing due to muscle tremor and slight patient movement. We will discuss artifact in more detail in Chapter 4. Remember that the artifact filter will correct only the printed output. If the computer performs interpretation, it will interpret the results from the actual nonfiltered information from the patient, not what is printed or viewed on the screen. This could cause inaccurate interpretation by the computer, which is why it is essential that a physician as well as the computer should interpret all ECGs.

LCD display

There are various other controls on the ECG machine that the user can set or use to enter information. For example, the user can enter data about the patient to be included on the printout along with the ECG results. This information would be entered into the LCD (liquid crystal diode) display (see Figure 3-9). This is the area of the machine where you can view the patient information you have entered. It is also where information from the ECG's computer is displayed. For example, a newer machine can detect if the arm leads or chest leads are reversed, and it will display this information in the LCD panel.

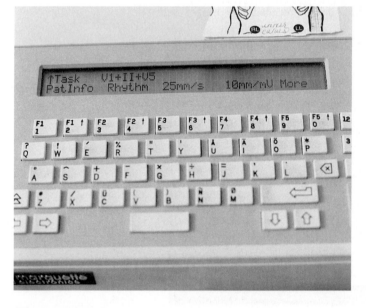

Figure 3-9: On newer ECG machines, information is entered into the LCD display. Some machines can even identify incorrect lead placement.

Heart rate limits

If the ECG machine has computer interpretation, the user may be able to set the heart rate limits. In other words, the operator can set the heart rate that the machine

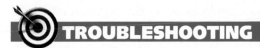
When the deflections on the ECG tracing are too short or tall, you will need to correct the gain. Be certain the machine is standardized correctly and then adjust the gain control if necessary.

will interpret as too slow (**bradycardia**) or too fast (**tachycardia**). If the heart rate is above or below the number set, the machine will indicate this by sounding an alarm and marking on the tracing.

Stylus and standardization control

Older ECG machines write on special paper with a heated **stylus.** The stylus reacts with the treated paper and produces a tracing. When the heat is turned up, a darker tracing results; when the heat is turned down, it produces a light tracing. The heat should be set so the tracing is clear and not too dark to avoid smearing or bleeding. Machines with a stylus must be standardized before use.

If you are using a machine that requires **standardization,** this procedure must be done in order to ensure that the machine is recording correctly. On most machines, pressing the standardization control produces a standardization mark. The stylus should move up 10 small squares and remain there for two small squares. If this does not occur, the machine must be adjusted before use. To make this adjustment, check the manufacturer's directions for the machine you are using.

Newer digital machines use thermal technology, which is achieved by heating dots as the paper moves across the print head. Digital machines require no manual standardization; the machine makes the adjustments automatically.

Lead selector

Most 12-lead ECG machines record each of the leads automatically. However, a lead selector is used to run each lead individually in case one or more leads needs to be repeated.

Electrodes and Electrolyte Products

Electrodes are sensors that are placed on a person's skin to pick up the electrical activity of the heart and conduct it to the ECG machine. The standard 12-lead ECG uses 10 electrodes. These electrodes come in a variety of types and can be reusable or disposable.

Plate

Reusable electrodes

Reusable electrodes include plates and bulbs (see Figure 3-10). Both types of reusable electrodes require special conduction materials. Conduction materials are electrolyte products that allow the electrical impulses to be recorded through the skin. These materials can be gels, pastes, or moistened flannel pads. They all contain an electrolyte solution, which provides an improved ECG tracing. When using electrolyte products such as gels and pastes, be sure to use the same amount for each electrode. Unequal amounts may cause poor recording. Electrolyte pads are the easiest to use. Unlike pastes and gels, they are not as messy, and each pad contains exactly the same amount of electrolyte solution. Electrolyte pads can also be

Bulb

Figure 3-10: Reusable electrodes are usually metal plates or bulbs. They must be cleaned after each ECG.

used to prepare the skin prior to placement of the electrodes. Reusable electrodes should be washed after each use and scoured with kitchen cleanser when necessary (about once a week). Excessive corrosion or an accumulation of electrolytes may also cause poor recording.

Disposable electrodes

Disposable electrodes are used more commonly because they reduce the possibility of cross-contamination and can be simply removed and discarded for easier cleanup (see Figure 3-11). The self-adhesive types stick easily to the patient's body. The gel is already applied so the electrodes will properly conduct the electrical impulses.

Each disposable electrode is normally used on only one ECG. The only exception occurs when a second ECG is performed on the same patient immediately after the first and the electrodes are not disturbed. If the electrodes stay on the patient's skin any longer than two sequential readings, the gel will dry out, resulting in inaccurate ECG tracings.

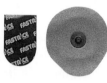

Figure 3-11: Disposable electrodes come in various shapes and sizes. Electrolyte gel or paste is not necessary since it is already contained on these electrodes.

For hospitalized patients, longer-lasting silver electrodes are now available. These electrodes are used for patients who require multiple and frequent ECGs (serial ECGs). When serial ECGs are required, it is important to ensure the same lead placement for each. A slight change often causes a change in the tracing. The silver electrodes are kept on the patient and checked daily.

No matter what type of electrode is used, they must be handled and stored correctly. If a package contains more electrodes than needed, the remaining electrodes must be kept in a sealed plastic bag so the gel will not dry out. Always check the expiration date on the package before use. Make sure the electrode gel has not dried out on any electrode. Even new electrodes should be checked before placement.

ECG Graph Paper

The ECG machine records an image of the heart's electrical activity onto graph paper. This image is the ECG waveform, or a series of waves and complexes recorded from the activity in the heart. The graph paper provides increments to measure the electrical activity produced on the tracing. Understanding the ECG paper is a necessary part of performing an ECG and is essential to interpreting the ECG (see Figure 3-12).

The two most commonly used types of paper are standard grid and dot matrix. Both are heat and pressure sensitive. Because the paper is pressure sensitive, you should handle it carefully to avoid marking it. Marks on the paper could make the tracing difficult to read or inaccurate. In addition, certain substances such as alcohol, plastic, sunlight,

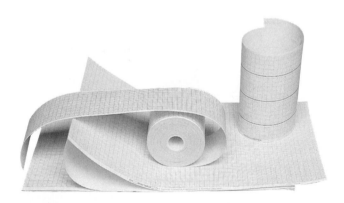

Figure 3-12: Choose the right size and type of graph paper for the ECG machine you will be using.

TROUBLESHOOTING

Handle and store the ECG report with care. It can be damaged easily, and if damaged, it cannot be interpreted by the physician.

and X-ray film can erase the tracing. Once the ECG is completed, it should be stored away from these substances. Some companies offer recording paper that requires no special handling or storage. This paper guarantees that the tracing will last for up to 50 years.

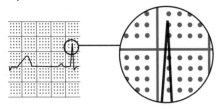 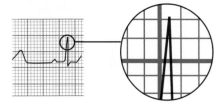

Figure 3-13: Comparison of ECG graph paper: dot matrix paper (left) requires less ink, is easier to read, and produces sharper photocopies, whereas standard grid paper (right) is slightly less expensive.

Dot matrix paper has some advantages over standard grid paper. Dot matrix reports require less ink, are easier to read, and produce sharper photocopies. One advantage of standard grid paper is that it is slightly less expensive (see Figure 3-13).

The standard paper speed for the ECG machine is 25 mm/sec. Be sure your ECG machine is set at this speed unless ordered otherwise. If you run the machine at any speed other than 25 mm/sec, be certain to note this on the ECG results. Prior to performing an ECG, make sure the machine has enough paper to record the results. Each machine has a paper loading procedure that you should become familiar with. Many of the machines warn you when the paper is nearly gone by making a red mark across the bottom of the tracing (see Figure 3-14). Read the manufacturer's directions for specific instructions on how to change the ECG machine paper. Keep a supply of paper on the ECG cart in case you run out of paper in the patient's room or examination room.

Figure 3-14: The thick line at the bottom of the ECG graph paper indicates that the paper needs to be changed.

Measurements

The ECG graph paper consists of precisely spaced horizontal and vertical lines. The horizontal readings represent time, measured in millimeters (mm). The vertical readings measure voltage, indicated in millivolts (mV). The heavy lines form boxes that are 5 mm by 5 mm in size. The smallest box on the graph paper represents .04 seconds in time and 1 mm or .1 mV in voltage. At the normal paper speed, one second equals 25 mm, or five heavy lines. Therefore, each vertical heavy line represents 0.20 of a second. Two large boxes represent 10 mm, which equals one centimeter (cm). ECG machines must be calibrated so that 1 cm = 1 mV. Each heavy line horizontally represents 5 mm or .5 mV (see Figure 3-15).

LAW AND ETHICS - Handling the ECG paper and report correctly is essential, since the ECG report is part of a patient's medical records and must be maintained for at least seven years.

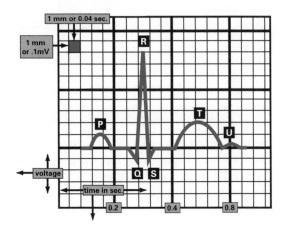

Five vertical heavy lines or boxes = 1 second

One vertical heavy line or box = 0.2 seconds

Smallest vertical line or box = 0.04 seconds

Two large horizontal heavy lines or boxes = 1 mV

Figure 3-15: ECG waveform with graph paper measurements

Table 3-2 **Calculating heart rates with measurement of the R to R interval**		
Large Boxes Between Two R Waves	Seconds Between Beats	Heart Beats per Minute
1	0.2	300
2	0.4	150
3	0.6	100
4	0.8	75
5	1.0	60
6	1.2	50

Figure 3-16: To estimate the heart rate with the R-R wave method, count the number of large boxes between two R waves and divide into 300. In this figure there are four full boxes between the R waves for an estimated rate of 75.

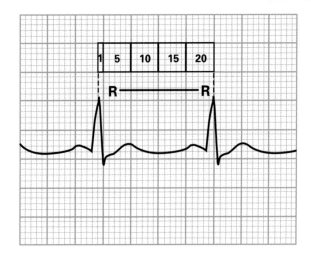

Calculating heart rate

When you are running the ECG at 25 mm/sec, there are 300 large boxes in a 1-minute strip. To determine the heart rate with a regular rhythm, you need to first determine the number of large boxes between two R waves on the ECG tracing. This number should be divided into 300. For example, if there were five boxes between the R waves, the heart rate would be 300 divided by 5, which equals 60 beats per minute. Table 3-2 provides the approximate heart rates based on this method of calculation. Also see Figure 3-16 for calculating heart rates using the R-R wave method.

Another method for estimating the heart rate is called the six-second method. First, identify a six-second section of the tracing. The ECG paper is usually marked at three-second intervals on the top or bottom of the strip with a vertical line. You will need to view 2 sections, or 30 boxes, horizontally. Second, count the number of complete complexes seen in one six-second interval. Each complex must include the P, QRS, and T wave. The complex should not be counted unless complete. Third, multiply the number of complexes by 10 to determine the estimated heart rate. This method can be used when the rhythm is irregular (see Figure 3-17).

Figure 3-17: To estimate the heart rate with the six-second method, locate a six-second section of the ECG rhythm strip (each small black line at the top of the strip indicates 15 boxes or three seconds), count the number of complete complexes in this section, then multiply the number of complexes by 10. In this figure, 8 complete complexes equal an estimated heart rate of 80.

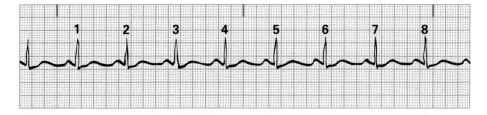

TROUBLESHOOTING

When calculating the heart rate by counting the complexes in the six-second interval, count the complete complexes only. If there is a portion of a complex at each end of the six-second section you are using, find another section on the tracing to view. Never count incomplete complexes; this will make your results inaccurate.

Chapter Review

The Match Game: Match the name of each of the following leads with their lead type. Place the correct letter on the line provided.

_____ **1.** V1

_____ **2.** aVR

_____ **3.** lead I

_____ **4.** lead II

_____ **5.** aVL

_____ **6.** V3

_____ **7.** V4

_____ **8.** V6

_____ **9.** aVF

_____ **10.** lead III

_____ **11.** V2

_____ **12.** V5

a. Standard limb lead
b. Augmented lead
c. Precordial lead

Match these terms related to the ECG with their definitions. Place the correct letter on the line provided.

_____ **13.** single-channel

_____ **14.** speed

_____ **15.** input

_____ **16.** gain

_____ **17.** lead

_____ **18.** multichannel

_____ **19.** mV

_____ **20.** mm

_____ **21.** signal processing

_____ **22.** electrode

_____ **23.** output display

a. disposable sensors that receive the electrical activity of the heart
b. changes the size of the ECG tracing
c. data that is entered into an ECG machine
d. indicates time on the ECG tracing
e. conductor wire attached to the ECG machine
f. ability to record more than one lead tracing at a time
g. indicates voltage on the ECG tracing
h. displays the tracing for the electrical activity of the heart
i. amplifies the electrical impulse and converts to mechanical action
j. records one lead tracing at a time
k. controls the speed of the paper during an ECG tracing

24. ECG machines have three basic functions. They are:

    a. input, signal processing, and output display

    b. input, standardization, and output display

    c. multichannel, single-channel, and signal processing

    d. standardization, input display and output display

25. To perform an ECG with accuracy the *best* source to obtain specific information about the machine is:

    a. the policy and procedure manual

    b. the manufacturer's directions

    c. your supervisor

    d. your textbook

26. The type of electrodes most commonly used are _____ and are used _____ .

    a. disposable, more than once

    b. reusable, more than once

    c. disposable, once

    d. reusable, once

27. What is the purpose of the LCD display?

    a. to allow entry and display of patient information

    b. to show the results of the ECG

    c. to sound alarms and errors

    d. to assist the patient to understand the procedure

28. What is the standard paper speed?

    a. 25 mm/sec

    b. 50 mm/sec

    c. .25 mm/sec

    d. .50 mm/sec

29. Which of the following is *not* a type of lead?

    a. standard

    b. augmented

    c. input

    d. precordial

30. The horizontal readings on the ECG paper represent _____ and the vertical readings represent _____ .

    a. voltage, time

    b. time, height

    c. time, voltage

    d. voltage, millivolts

Match the size of the line with the time on the tracing at 25mm/sec paper speed. Place your answer in the space provided.

_____ 31. 5 heavy lines or boxes

_____ 32. 1 vertical heavy line or box

_____ 33. smallest vertical line or box

a. 1 second
b. .04 second
c. .2 second

Match the lead wire and its color. Place your answer in the space provided.

_____ **34.** left leg (LL)

_____ **35.** right arm (RA)

_____ **36.** right leg (RL)

_____ **37.** left arm (LA)

a. green
b. white
c. black
d. red

Label the Parts

38. Label the lead tracings that produce the Einthoven triangle.

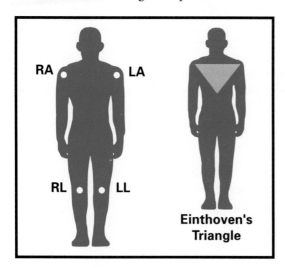
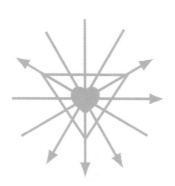

39. Label the measurements indicated on the following figure.

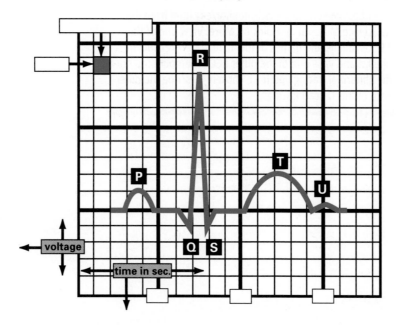

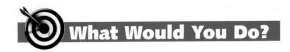 **What Would You Do?**

Read the following situations and use your critical thinking skills to determine how you would handle each. Write your answer in detail in the space provided.

40. When you start to take the ECG machine to a patient's room, you notice a red line along the bottom of the ECG paper. What should you do?

_____

41. When preparing to do an ECG, you find an open package of disposable electrodes on top of the ECG cart. Would you use these electrodes? Why or why not?

_____

42. You are preparing to attach the electrodes and lead wires for a 12-lead ECG. You are unable to read the letters on each of the lead wires. You place the electrodes and lead wires, but when you run the tracing it looks like a bunch of scratches. What do you think the problem is and how would you solve it?

_____

43. When performing a 12-lead ECG, you notice that the tracing line is very thick and hard to view. In addition, one of the leads does not record properly. What would you do?

_____

 GET CONNECTED TO THE WEB

Go to the Website http://www.fi.edu/biosci/monitor/ekg.html from the Franklin Institute Science Museum and click on More. View one of the normal 12-lead ECGs and list the names of the 12-lead tracings shown. Now return to the list and view one of the other ECGs. Compare the normal ECG with the abnormal tracing you have chosen. Describe the differences seen in each of the 12-lead tracings.

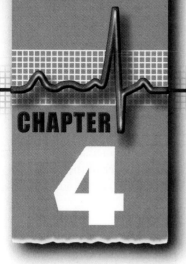

4

Performing an ECG

Objectives

Upon completion of the chapter, you should be able to:

▶ Demonstrate proficiency in preparing the patient, room, and equipment for an ECG

▶ Discuss what to do in the event that the patient refuses an ECG

▶ Demonstrate the proper procedure for the application of the electrodes and lead wires for a 12-lead ECG

▶ Identify at least three ways to maintain infection control during the ECG procedure

▶ Identify at least three ways to provide for safety during the ECG procedure

▶ Identify types of artifact and how to prevent or correct them

▶ Demonstrate the proper procedure for recording and reporting a 12-lead ECG

▶ Mount a single-lead ECG tracing correctly

▶ Compare and contrast the adult and pediatric ECG procedure

▶ Troubleshoot special patient circumstances when performing an ECG

▶ Clean and care for the ECG equipment

Key Terms

AC (alternating current) interference - Unwanted markings on the ECG caused by other electrical current sources.

angle of Louis - A ridge about an inch or so below the suprasternal notch where the main part of the sternum and the top of the sternum, known as the manubrium, are attached.

anterior axillary line - An imaginary vertical line starting at the edge of the chest where the armpit begins.

artifact - Unwanted marks on the ECG tracing caused by activity other than the heart's electrical activity.

complexes - Atrial or ventricular contractions as they appear on the ECG; complete ECG waveforms.

dextrocardia - A congenital defect where the left ventricle, left atrium, aortic arch, and stomach are located on the right side of the chest.

Key Terms (cont.)

intercostal space (ICS) - The space between two ribs.

midaxillary line - An imaginary vertical line that starts at the middle of the armpit.

midclavicular line - An imaginary line on the chest that runs vertically through the center of the clavicle.

seizure - An interruption of the electrical activity in the brain that causes involuntary muscle movement and sometimes unconsciousness.

somatic tremor - Voluntary or involuntary muscle movement; also known as body tremor.

stat - Immediately.

suprasternal notch - The dip you feel at the base of the neck just above where the clavicle attaches to the sternum.

wandering baseline - When the tracing of an ECG drifts away from the center of the paper; also called baseline shift. It has many causes, which can be corrected.

Now that you understand how the ECG is used, the anatomy of the heart, and the electrocardiograph, the next step is to record an ECG. The ECG experience should be pleasant to the patient and not produce anxiety. The ECG procedure must be done correctly and the tracing must be accurate. This chapter will provide you with information necessary to record an ECG professionally, without error, while keeping the patient as comfortable as possible.

Preparation for the ECG Procedure

Prior to performing the ECG you will need to prepare the room. Certain conditions in the room where the ECG is to be performed should be considered. For example electrical currents in the room can interfere with the tracing. If possible, choose a room away from other electrical equipment and X-ray machines. If electrical equipment is in the room, turn off any that you can during the tracing. The ECG machine should be placed away from other sources of electrical currents such as wires or cords.

An ECG must be ordered by a physician and an order form must be completed prior to the procedure. This form may be called a requisition or consult and should be placed in the patient's record. It should include why the ECG was ordered and the following identifying information:

- Patient name and identification number
- Location, date, and time of recording
- Patient age, sex, race, and cardiac medications
- Weight and height
- Any special condition or position of the patient during the recording

If this information is not included on the requisition or consult, you should ask the patient or find the information in the patient's record.

Many facilities have computerized billing systems. The ECG order is frequently entered through this system. Entering the patient identifying information into the computer will produce the order form and generate patient charges. If your facility does not have a computer system, the information should be handwritten on the order form, consult, or requisition, whichever your facility uses.

The patient identifying information should also be entered through the LCD panel on the ECG machine prior to the recording. If the ECG machine does not allow you to enter the information, you should write it on the completed ECG. Most importantly, all information should be

PATIENT EDUCATION AND COMMUNICATION - Certain cardiac medications can change the ECG tracing. Determine if your patient is on any cardiac medications prior to the ECG procedure, and if so, inform the physician and write the names of the medications on the ECG report.

written or entered accurately no matter what type of ECG machine or order system you are using.

Before beginning the procedure, make sure the ECG machine has a good supply of paper loaded in it. If a red line is seen across the bottom of the last tracing, you should place fresh paper in the ECG machine before beginning. This should be done prior to taking the ECG machine to the room with the patient. Before opening the new paper, look on the package for loading instructions. Since ECG machines and paper differ, this is a valuable source of information.

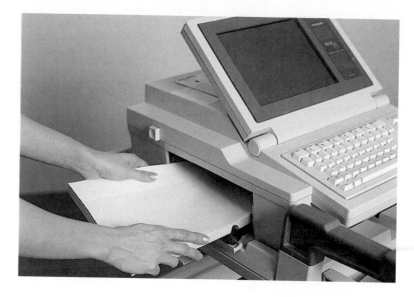

Figure 4-1: Make sure the ECG paper is properly loaded and aligned before recording an ECG.

Typically, the single-channel ECG machines use a thin roll and multichannel ECG machines use wider, fan-folded type paper. Each ECG machine will have a release button or lever that will open the ECG equipment for the paper to be inserted. Place the paper inside the machine correctly. Thread it through the roller to the outside of the machine and align. Close the paper-loading compartment and run the machine to check for proper functioning and alignment (see Figure 4-1).

Communicating with the Patient

Always identify the patient before performing any procedure by stating the patient's full name. Check the name on the patient's identification band, if available. If the patient is unable to respond and has no identification band, you should confirm the identity with a family member or other health care professional caring for the patient.

Introduce yourself and explain what you are about to do. State "I am going to perform an electrocardiogram on you today. Have you ever had an ECG done before?" Stating both ECG and electrocardiogram helps the patient relate that they are the same. If the patient has not had an ECG, explain the procedure in more detail. Assure the patient that the procedure is harmless and painless. Avoid using words that may frighten the patient such as electricity or wires. Patients, particularly children, who have not had an ECG before may be afraid of the machine and wires. The patient should be relaxed and comfortable. Maintaining a calm, competent manner and answering the patient's questions will help the patient relax.

If the patient refuses an ECG, determine the cause of the refusal. Some people may have fear or concern about the procedure. Provide any information or reassurance the patient may need. Frequently, patients see the wires and think the machine will shock them. Be sure you explain carefully that you are only going to measure the electricity that is already inside their body. If the patient still refuses, notify your supervisor.

In preparing for an ECG, the patient should remove any clothing above the waist. Provide the patient with a drape, such as a sheet or blanket. The patient may also wear a hospital-type gown with the opening in the front. The patient should remove any jewelry that would interfere with the electrode placement or touch the electrodes. This may include necklaces, watches, bracelets, or ankle bracelets. The patient should be

LAW AND ETHICS - The ECG is part of the medical record. Enter the patient information thoroughly and accurately. Remember, the patient's medical record can be used as part of a medical professional liability case.

PATIENT EDUCATION AND COMMUNICATION - Remember, even if a patient is not able to respond, he or she may still hear you. Always explain the procedure before beginning the ECG.

positioned as comfortably as possible on his or her back and should remain relaxed and still throughout the procedure. To ensure comfort, place a small pillow under the patient's head and an extra pillow under the knees, if preferred.

The position of the patient is important during an ECG. Expose the patient's chest and extremities where you will be placing the leads. If possible, work from the left side of the bed or exam table, since most of the electrodes and leads are placed on the left side of the chest. Ensure that the arms and legs are supported on the exam table or bed. Take care to provide for privacy by using the blanket or sheet to drape the patient. It is especially important to drape a female patient's breasts for comfort and to prevent embarrassment. A sheet or blanket will also keep the patient warm and prevent chills. Chills may produce shivers that could interfere with the tracing. Make sure that the bed or exam table is not touching the wall or any electrical equipment and that the patient is not touching any metal.

Identifying Anatomical Landmarks

Once you have properly positioned the patient on the bed or exam table, you will need to place the electrodes on the chest and limbs. In order to place the chest electrodes for the ECG, you must have an understanding of the anatomy and certain landmarks on the chest. Each lead, V1 to V6, must be placed on the correct site on the chest. These sites can be identified by knowing the underlying bones and a set of imaginary lines on the exterior of the chest.

The bones of the chest include the clavicle, the sternum, and the ribs. The imaginary lines include the midclavicular line, the midaxillary line, and the anterior axillary line. On most patients, the **midclavicular line** starts in the center of the clavicle and passes vertically through the nipple line. The **anterior axillary line** starts in the front of the axilla and runs down the left side of the chest. The **midaxillary line** starts in the middle of the axilla (armpit) and runs down the side of the chest.

Other sites on the chest you must be able to locate include the intercostal spaces, suprasternal notch, and the angle of Louis. To feel the **intercostal space** (ICS), or space between two ribs, locate the sternum. Press your fingers to the edge of the sternum on the left or right side. The outer edge of the sternum is known as the sternal border. Between each connected rib you should feel a dip or dent. Feeling as close to the sternal border as possible will make it easier. The **suprasternal notch** is the dip you feel at the base of the neck just above where the clavicle attaches to the sternum. The **angle of Louis** is a ridge about an inch or so below the suprasternal notch. It is where the main part of the sternum and the manubrium (top of the sternum) attach (see Figure 4-2).

Figure 4-2: Anatomical landmarks for chest lead placement

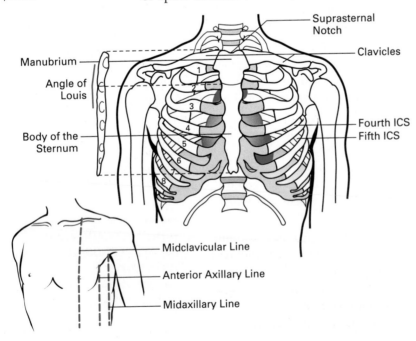

Suprasternal Notch

Clavicles

Manubrium

Angle of Louis

Body of the Sternum

Fourth ICS

Fifth ICS

Midclavicular Line

Anterior Axillary Line

Midaxillary Line

Applying the Electrodes and Leads

Before applying the electrodes on the chest, make sure the skin at the sites is clean and dry. Remove any lotion or oil from the skin with gauze and alcohol or an alcohol swab. You may use electrolyte pads to prep the skin. If the patient has a great deal of chest hair, you may also need to shave small areas of the chest so the electrodes will adhere to the skin properly. When placing electrodes for continuous monitoring, you should clip the hair instead of shaving. This prevents the patient from scratching the electrode site as the hair grows in (see Table 4-1).

When applying chest lead V1, locate the fourth intercostal space at the right sternal border. The fourth intercostal space is the dent you feel between the fourth and fifth ribs. V2 should be placed at the fourth intercostal space on the left sternal border. Skip V3 and place V4 next. V4 is placed at the fifth intercostal space on the left midclavicular line. Locate the site of the intersection between the fifth ICS and the midclavicular line. In most people, this site is directly below the nipple. Now place V3 midway between V2 and V4. Skip V5 and place V6 next, directly in line with V4 on the midaxillary line. Place V5 midway between V4 and V6 on the left anterior axillary line (see Figure 4-3 and Table 4-2 on p. 54).

The procedure is the same when placing the chest electrodes on a female. If the patient has large breasts, simply lift the left breast and place the electrodes in the closest position possible. Leads V4 and V5 will be the most affected. Avoid placing the electrodes directly on breast tissue since it is a poor conductor of electricity.

The limb electrodes are placed on the wrists or upper arms and the inside of the lower legs. You should pick a fleshy area with the least amount of hair. If the placement of the arm leads on the patient's wrists is not possible due to injury, amputation, IV placement, casts, or otherwise, you should chose a different site. The alternate site of placement for arm leads is on the shoulders. The leads should be placed on the same site on each arm and should match. For example, if a patient has a cast or an IV on the left wrist, you will need to move *both* left and right electrodes to the shoulders.

Table 4-1 Applying leads correctly

- Choose a flat, nonmuscular area.
- Use the flat, fleshy area just above the wrists and ankles for the limb leads.
- Alternate sites include the upper arms near the shoulders and upper legs.
- Prep the skin with an electrolyte pad, if available.
- When necessary, cleanse the electrode sites with an alcohol pad or mild soap and water.
- Dry the skin completely before applying the electrodes.
- Shave the hair from the site only if necessary.
- Clip the hair, instead of shaving, when applying continuous monitor leads.

SAFETY AND INFECTION CONTROL - During the ECG procedure, raise the safety rail on the opposite side of the bed or exam table from where you are working, if available.

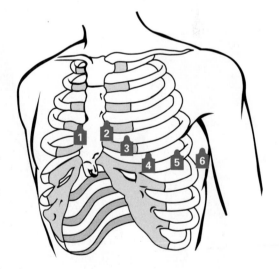

Figure 4-3: Chest lead placement

TROUBLESHOOTING

When locating the midclavicular line for chest lead placement, keep in mind that the midclavicular line does not always run directly through the nipple line. This is most often the case with obese patients or females with large breasts.

Identifying Lead Wires

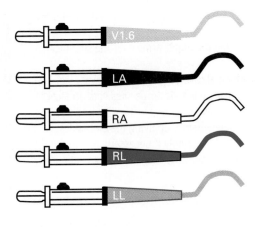

RA = right arm   ○ **White**
LA = left arm   ● **Black**
RL = right leg   ◉ **Green**
LL = left leg   ◉ **Red**
V1 to V6 = chest leads ○ **Brown**

Figure 4-4: Color and letter coding identify the lead wires for an ECG machine.

Table 4-2 **Chest lead placement**
V1 - fourth intercostal space, right sternal border
V2 - fourth intercostal space, left sternal border
V3 - halfway between V2 and V4
V4 - fifth intercostal space at the midclavicular line
V5 - on the same horizontal level with V4, at the anterior axillary line
V6 - on the same horizontal level with V4 and V5, at the midaxillary line

When placement of the leg leads on the patient's lower legs or ankles is not possible, the alternate site for placement is on the upper legs. They should be placed as close to the trunk as possible. This may be necessary when a patient is an amputee or has an injury or bandage on one of the lower legs. The leads should be placed at the same site on each leg: if you place one lead above the knee on the left, then the right leg lead should also be placed above the knee.

After all of the electrodes have been properly positioned, you must attach the lead cable wires. Identify the correct cable for each electrode based on color and letter abbreviations. For example, the chest leads are usually brown and are marked V1 to V6 (see Figure 4-4). The correct cable must be attached to the corresponding electrode to ensure an accurate tracing. With most ECG machines, the limb leads should be pointed toward the hands and feet when placed on the electrodes. Chest electrodes are usually pointed toward the head but may be pointed toward the feet; check the manufacturer's directions. The electrodes should be secure and the lead wires should be supported.

The ECG lead wire cables should follow the contours of the body when attached to the ECG electrodes. Avoid looping the wires outside of the body and check each wire once it is connected to ensure that there is no tension on the electrodes or leads (see Figure 4-5).

Lead Wires
○ White
● Black
◉ Brown
◉ Red
◉ Green

Figure 4-5: Correct (left) and incorrect (right) lead cable placement. Avoid looping the wires outside the body and check each wire once it is connected to ensure that there is no tension on the electrodes or leads.

Safety and Infection Control

When performing an ECG you must always follow precautions. You must practice Universal Precautions at all times. Universal Precautions, as discussed in Chapter 2, are followed in all situations in which job exposure to blood or body fluids is likely. Wash your hands carefully before the procedure to prevent transfer of microorganisms. Wear gloves if there is a risk of exposure to the patient's blood or other body fluids.

In the hospital you will need to follow Standard Precautions for patients in isolation. Depending on the type of isolation, masks, eye protection, and gowns may also be necessary when entering the room. Follow the facility's policy and the guidelines provided in Table 4-3. You should know Standard Precautions related to all hospitalized patients and maintain them throughout the procedure. As a rule, it is better to wear gloves even if it is not necessary. Do not forget to wash your hands before putting on the gloves and after removing them.

PATIENT EDUCATION AND COMMUNICATION - When moving the electrodes to a different location due to an amputation or bandages, you should document this on the 12-lead ECG recording.

Table 4-3 Infection control guidelines for isolation of hospitalized patients

In addition to Standard Precautions, follow these guidelines and the policy of your place of employment to prevent the spread of infections.

Airborne precautions

For patients known or suspected to be infected with microorganisms transmitted by minute airborne droplets:
- Use a private room that has monitored negative air.
- Keep the room door closed and the patient in the room.
- Wear respiratory protection when entering the room of a patient with known or suspected infectious pulmonary tuberculosis.
- Wear special HEPA or N-95 masks when entering the room.
- Do not enter the room of a patient known or suspected to have rubeola or varicella if you are susceptible: if you must enter the room, wear respiratory protection.
- Limit the movement and transport of patients from the room to essential purposes only.
- Place a surgical mask on the patient, if transport or movement is necessary.

Droplet precautions

For patients known or suspected to be infected with microorganisms transmitted by droplets that can be generated by the patient during coughing, sneezing, talking, or the performance of procedures:
- Place patient in a private room (special air handling and ventilation are not necessary and the door may remain open).
- Wear a mask when working within 3 feet of the patient.
- Limit the movement and transport of the patient from the room to essential purposes only.
- Use a mask on the patient, if transport or movement is necessary.

Contact precautions

For patients known or suspected to be infected or colonized with microorganisms that can be transmitted by direct or indirect contact (direct contact includes hand or skin-to-skin contact that occurs when performing patient care that requires touching the patient's dry skin; indirect contact includes touching environmental surfaces or patient-care items in the patient's environment):
- Place patients in a private room.
- Wear gloves according to Standard (or Universal) Precautions.
- Wear gloves when entering the room and while providing patient care.
- Change gloves after having contact with infective material that may contain high concentrations of microorganisms such as feces and wound drainage.
- Remove gloves before leaving the patient's room.
- Wash hands immediately.
- Do not touch potentially contaminated environmental surfaces or items in the patient's room after glove removal.

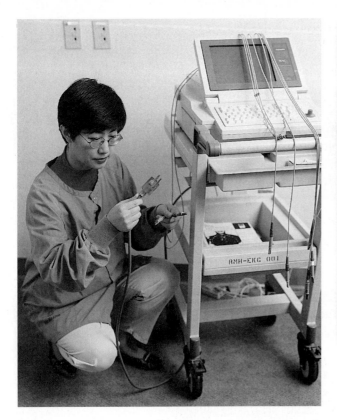

Figure 4-6: Check the lead wires and electrical cord for breaks or fraying before using the ECG machine.

General safety guidelines and safety measures specific to the ECG procedure must also be practiced. Before beginning the procedure, you should raise the side rail on the unattended side of the patient's bed or exam table. If the patient is on an exam table, have them lie down and pull the extension out for their legs and feet. Prior to performing the ECG, check to be sure that the grounding prong is securely attached to the plug. Plug the machine in securely. Ensure that the bed or exam table is not touching the wall or any electrical equipment. Be sure that the patient is not touching the bed or exam table frame or safety rail. Always check the insulation on the lead wires for cracks before each use (see Table 4-4 and Figure 4-6).

When you have finished the procedure, provide for the patient's safety and comfort. Assist him or her to a comfortable position in which to dress. After the procedure, you should clean the lead wires, leads, and machine. If you performed an ECG on a patient in isolation or with a contagious disease, you will need to clean the equipment properly to prevent the spread of infection. Observe the guidelines at your place of employment and the manufacturer's directions for the correct cleaning technique. Once you have completed the entire procedure, including cleanup, you should wash your hands.

Operating the ECG Machine

SAFETY AND INFECTION CONTROL - Check the grounding prong, the power cord, and the insulation on the lead wires for cracks and fraying each time you perform an ECG. If the cord or lead wires are damaged, replace immediately before performing the ECG.

Before operating the ECG machine, make sure you have done the following:

- Identify and communicate with the patient
- Prepare the patient and the room
- Provide for safety and infection control
- Locate and check the equipment for functioning
- Load the ECG graph paper
- Attach the electrodes and leads

Now you should be ready to operate the ECG machine. For an automatic ECG, simply press the Run or Auto button. Check the LCD display for errors. If the ECG machine provides interpretation, it will print out along with the tracing. This process takes only about 15-20 seconds.

For a manual ECG machine make sure the equipment is standardized and set to lead I. You may need to run a few **complexes** (complete ECG waveforms) and then insert a standardization mark using the standardization control discussed in Chapter 3. The mark should be set between the T wave of one complex and the P wave of the next. Follow specific directions provided in the operator's manual.

Table 4-5 Manual coding for the ECG leads

When using a single-channel ECG machine that does not mark the lead names, you can use the dot and dash codes shown here. A marker button on the machine can be tapped to make the corresponding marks on the ECG tracing. Newer machines mark the lead tracings automatically.

Lead	Mark	Lead	Mark
I	.	V1	-.
II	..	V2	-..
III	...	V3	-...
aVR	-	V4	-....
aVL	--	V5	-.....
aVF	---	V6	-......

Some ECG machines automatically mark the lead codes. If the equipment you are using does not, mark each code manually during the tracing. While the ECG is running, change the lead code dial, then mark each lead (see Table 4-5). You should run about 8 to10 inches of complexes for leads I, II, and III. For the rest of the leads, 5 inches should be sufficient. Identify the recording with the patient's name, the date, and other required information. You will need to mount the tracing immediately upon completion of the ECG. Mounting the ECG will be discussed later in this chapter under "Reporting ECG Results."

Checking the ECG Tracing

Certain problems can occur when obtaining an ECG tracing. The most frequent problem is unwanted marks on the ECG. These marks are called **artifact.** The marks are not caused by the heart activity; they are caused by some other source of movement or electrical activity. When an ECG tracing has these unwanted marks, it is difficult or impossible to read. You are responsible for producing a correct tracing without artifact. In order to do this, you must first recognize artifact and then be able to eliminate it. The three most common causes are somatic tremor, wandering baseline; and AC interference (see Table 4-6 on p. 58).

Somatic tremor

Sometimes a patient's muscles will move, either voluntarily or involuntarily, which can produce **somatic tremor,** also known as body tremor. Movement of the muscles of the body is controlled by electrical voltages. These voltages are erratic, unlike the cardiac voltage, which is consistent. Somatic tremor appears as large erratic spikes on the ECG tracing (see Figure 4-7).

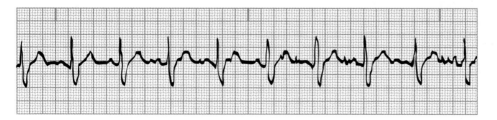

Figure 4-7: Somatic tremor appears as large erratic spikes on the ECG tracing.

Table 4-6 Correcting artifact

Type of Artifact	Specific Problem	Correction
Somatic tremor	Involuntary muscle movement: shivering, muscle tension, pain, fear	Reassure the patient, warm the patient, and encourage him or her to take slow, deep breaths
	Voluntary movement: talking, chewing gum	Remind the patient not to make any movement during the procedure
	Movement due to neuromuscular disorder such as Parkinson's disease	Have the patient put his or her hands, palms down, under the buttocks
Wandering baseline	Improperly applied electrodes	Apply electrodes securely, make sure that the entire surface is in contact with the patient's skin
	Pulling on electrodes from unsupported lead wires	Remove tension from lead wires
	Old, corroded, or dirty electrodes	Keep reusable electrodes clean; store unused disposable ones in plastic bags
	Oil, lotion, or dirt on the skin under the electrodes	Clean the skin with alcohol and gauze or an alcohol prep pad
	Too little or dried out electrode gel	Use new disposable electrodes and store unused ones in a plastic bag; if using gel, apply plenty of new solution to electrodes
Alternating current (AC) interference	Improper grounding	Ensure that the plug has three prongs and is plugged into a grounded electrical outlet
	Other electrical equipment	Unplug equipment and wait until any other procedure is done, if possible
	Lead wires crossed and not pointed toward the hands and feet	Reposition the lead wires and ensure that they follow limbs and are pointed toward the hands and feet
	Electrical wiring in the walls or ceiling	Move the patient's bed away from the wall
	Corroded or dirty leads	Clean the leads after each use

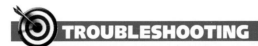

TROUBLESHOOTING

If your hospitalized patient requires daily ECGs for comparison by the physician, the ECG tracing may look different if the electrodes are placed in different sites on the chest and limbs. Each time you record an ECG on the patient, place the leads on the same site or as close as possible to the placement from the previous ECG.

Voluntary muscle movements are due to tension, fear, gum chewing, talking, uncomfortable position, or pain. They may also be due to shivering or tense muscles. You should identify the correct cause before proceeding with the ECG. Knowing the cause will help you eliminate the artifact. Warm or reassure the patient if he or she is cold or frightened. Encourage slow, deep breaths to help calm the patient. Remind the patient to refrain from moving or talking.

Sometimes involuntary muscle movements are due to Parkinson's disease or other neuromuscular disorders. These are more difficult to control. Have patients who suffer from neuromuscular disorders put their hands, palms down, under their buttocks. This will decrease the tremor and improve the tracing. If a patient has this type of tremor, it should be recorded on the ECG tracing.

Wandering baseline (baseline shift)

Wandering baseline, or baseline shift, occurs when the tracing drifts away from the center of the graph paper (see Figure 4-8). Baseline shift can have many causes. Typically, it is due to improper electrode application such as the following:

- too loose or incorrect electrode application
- tension or pulling on electrode lead wires
- too little electrode gel or solution
- old or dried out electrode gel or solution
- corroded or dirty electrodes
- oil, lotion, or dirt under the electrodes

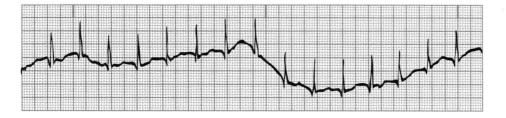

Figure 4-8: Wandering baseline occurs when the baseline of the ECG tracing drifts away from the center of the ECG graph paper.

To avoid problems with wandering baseline, apply the electrodes securely and make sure they are not too loose or tight. Be certain that the entire surface is in contact with the patient's skin. Check the lead wires and remove any tension from them. Use fresh electrode gel or new disposable electrodes. Make sure that previously opened electrodes have been stored in a plastic bag or container. Clean the leads after each use. Clean the patient's skin carefully before applying electrodes.

TROUBLESHOOTING

If you are using a newer multichannel 12-lead ECG machine you usually do not have to mark the tracing or run a certain amount of paper for each lead. The machine will automatically run all 12 leads and identify the code for each lead.

Alternating current (AC) interference

AC current is normally present in all electrical equipment. Sometimes the wires can radiate or leak a small amount of energy into the immediate surrounding area. When a patient is present in this area, the patient's body may pick up some of the current. This current is then registered on the ECG and is called **AC (alternating current) interference.** AC interference will appear as uniform small spikes on the ECG tracing (see Figure 4-9).

Figure 4-9: AC (alternating current) interference appears as uniform small spikes on the ECG tracing.

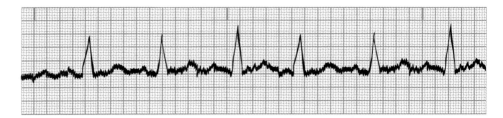

Many different things can cause AC interference artifact. These include improper grounding, other electrical equipment, lead wires crossed, and corroded or dirty electrodes. Eliminating the cause and using proper technique can prevent AC interference artifact. Eliminating sources of electrical current, ensuring proper grounding of the machine, and attaching the lead wires correctly can reduce AC interference.

The cause of AC interference is sometimes difficult to determine. You may still have AC interference even after you have checked that the machine is properly grounded, the lead wires are correct, and other equipment is turned off. In order to find the source, you can try this technique. Run lead I, lead II, and lead III and look for interference. Evaluate each strip for interference to determine the direction or source of interference (see Table 4-7). For example, if you have the most interference in leads II and III, the source is probably near or on the left arm. You may need to rotate the bed or exam table away from the source. You may just need to ground the bed by running a ground wire from the ECG machine to the bed. Also, do not forget the proper placement of the lead cables. They should follow the body contours. In addition, do not run the power cord under or over the bed or exam table. This is another possible source of electrical interference.

Artifact can also be caused by other sources. High-tension wires and transformers on a power pole and diathermy machines used to give high-frequency currents as heat treatments can cause AC interference. Electrocautery and X-ray machines can also interfere if they are in the room or an adjacent room. Even the electrical wires in the walls, ceiling, and floor, although they are not visible, can cause artifact. Some new ECG machines have a battery that allows you to unplug and still perform the ECG. Unplugging the machine eliminates any AC interference that may be produced from the electrical outlet.

Table 4-7 Troubleshooting AC interference

Leads with most AC interference noted	Source of interference or direction
Leads I and II	Right arm
Leads I and III	Left arm
Leads II and III	Left leg

🎯 TROUBLESHOOTING

If your patient is diaphoretic (sweating) and the electrodes will not stay attached during the monitoring or ECG tracing, consider cleaning the skin thoroughly and applying benzoin or spray deodorant to the site. Let the skin dry and then apply the electrodes.

> If a flat line without deflections occurs during the tracing, it could be asystole (indicates no heart beat). Remain calm and check the patient first, since the patient is your number one concern. If the patient is able to respond, check the electrodes, lead wires, and cables.

There are some additional problems you may encounter when obtaining an ECG. One example is an interrupted baseline on one or more leads. This appears as a flat line on the tracing. This could occur when a wire is not plugged in correctly or is loose. If a flat line occurs on more than one lead, it may be that the wires have been switched. Check your machine cables and connections. Ensure that the machine is set to obtain a tracing. Do not forget to check for loose or broken lead wires, which may also cause a break in the complexes or an interrupted baseline.

After troubleshooting any problem, if you cannot correct it, report it to your supervisor. If it is an AC interference problem, the biomedical engineering department, if available, may need to track down the source of the interference. It could also be that the machine requires service. In this case, the manufacturer should be called for information and assistance.

Reporting ECG results

When you have completed an ECG, use the method your facility requires for reporting the results. Check your facility policy to be certain you are placing the completed ECG tracings in the appropriate place. In many situations you will be required to make two copies, one to be placed on the patient's chart and the other to be read by the consulting physician. In the hospital the second copy is often taken back to the ECG laboratory, where it is placed in a special box or chart. The second copy may also be placed in a box at the nursing station where the patient is located. In an ambulatory care facility, it may be attached to the front of the chart and/or placed on the physician's desk.

Some facilities have a computer that can read the ECG electronically. In addition, sometimes ECG tracings are faxed to other locations. These procedures require special equipment. You may be asked to perform either of these procedures. If so, you must be trained using your facility's equipment. If the ECG was ordered **stat** (immediately), you will need to give the results directly and immediately to your superior. If your supervisor is not available, place the results on top of the chart, find your supervisor, and inform him or her that the ECG has been completed. Remember, in a stat situation the patient may have a condition that needs immediate treatment and no time should be wasted.

As previously discussed, billing is another issue to consider when reporting completion of an ECG. When you enter the data into the machine or on the designated form, it must be complete and accurate. If the patient is not charged for the procedure, this can have an adverse effect on the hospital's finances and subsequently your job. Check the facility policy to be certain you have completed the necessary steps to ensure that the patient will be charged.

In many facilities the information is entered into a computer to be sent to the billing department. You may need to enter the patient's diagnosis, which is provided by the physician and is found on the chart. Each diagnosis has a special diagnostic code, known as an ICD-9 code. In

SAFETY AND INFECTION CONTROL - Cleaning the ECG machine and maintaining the supplies are necessary for safe and efficient ECG recording and accurate tracings.

some cases, you will need to identify the correct code when entering the information for the billing department. Using these codes helps ensure that the facility is reimbursed for the procedure.

Mounting the ECG tracing

Single-channel ECG machines produce tracings on a single narrow strip displaying each of the 12 leads. When the tracing is recorded, each of the 12 leads should be marked so you will be able to identify them. If you are using a single-channel machine, you will need to mount the tracing so it can be evaluated. Most companies have standard mounts that require you to identify each lead and place it in the appropriate position on the mount. The single tracing can be cut into smaller segments to place on the preprinted mount. In addition, you will need to record on the mount identifying information and any special patient circumstances of the ECG procedure. Following proper mounting procedure is vital to ensure that the physician can easily review and interpret the results (see Figure 4-10).

Figure 4-10: Single-channel ECG tracings must be cut into smaller segments and placed onto a cardboard mount for viewing and evaluation by the physician.

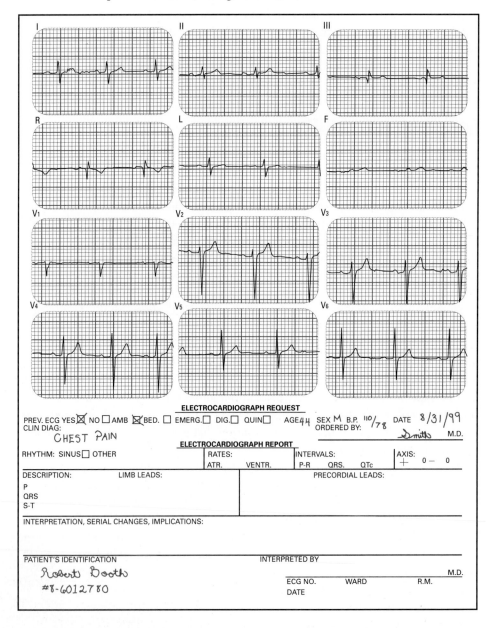

Equipment Maintenance

Care and maintenance of the ECG machine must be done and is your responsibility. Become familiar with the manufacturer's instructions for operation and maintenance of the ECG machine. The operator's manual for the machine you are using will include specific directions about routine care and maintenance. General day-to-day care and maintenance includes cleaning the ECG machine and stocking the supplies, such as electrodes, skin preparation, paper, and cleaning supplies.

Keep the ECG machine clean to prevent transmission of infection and to create a positive image of yourself and the facility where you are employed. Use a small amount of nonabrasive cleaner on the equipment case, cover, and control panel. Wipe the machine dry with a soft cloth. Follow the specific directions in the operator's manual for the disinfection procedure.

The cables and reusable electrodes should be disinfected frequently. Use a soft cloth moistened with disinfectant and wipe the entire cable and reusable electrode. You can also use packaged disinfectant wipes if they are available. Keep these available on the ECG cart. Do not place the cables in fluid or use heat sterilization. Do not use acetone, ether, or other harsh chemicals or solvents. Always follow the manufacturer's directions for best results.

Reusable electrodes require additional attention. After each use, wash the electrodes to prevent a build-up of gel or paste. Scour them once a week with an abrasive kitchen cleanser to prevent corrosion and restore the bright finish to the contact surfaces. Do not forget to clean the metal tips of the patient cable. Electrolyte gel or paste can build up on the metal tips and prevent proper contact with the electrodes. The electrode straps should be washed and checked for cracks. Replace any broken or cracked straps immediately.

When using disposable electrodes, carefully maintain the alligator clips used for attachment. Check them to ensure that the pins fit snugly on the electrode. Check for small amounts of electrolyte paste or gel that may cling to the clips. These bits of paste may prevent good contact with the electrodes (see Figure 4-11).

Wipe down the patient cables and lead wires with a damp cloth. Replace them neatly on the ECG machine for storage (see Figure 4-12). Inspect them regularly for cracks or fraying. Replace any cables that are damaged.

Figure 4-11: This newer type of alligator clip is frequently used for the ECG. Wipe these clips clean after use to prevent electrolyte gel or paste from getting stuck between the teeth of the clip.

Figure 4-12: When storing the ECG machine, place the lead wires and cables neatly over the machine. For safety, inspect each wire for cracks or fraying.

Pediatric ECG

When preparing a child for an ECG it is important to give simple directions that he or she can understand. Identify yourself and explain what you are going to do. Allow the child to ask questions. Avoid technical words like electrodes and electrocardiogram. Use the word "stickers" to describe electrodes. If the child is fearful of the "stickers," place them on a toy, doll, or parent. This will show the child that the procedure does not hurt. Explain that you are going to take a "picture" of the child's heart. Because children can usually identify with picture

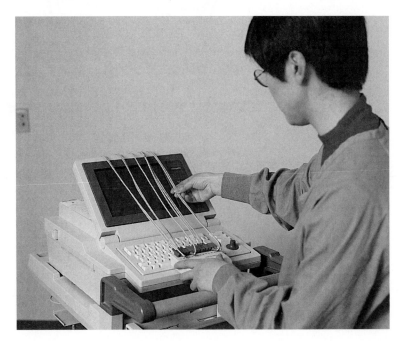

taking, this will help them understand that they need to be still during the "picture."

Always identify the child by name and check his or her identification armband. If the parents are present, you may allow them to stay. For a small child or infant, the parent can assist by letting the child lie quietly in their arms. A fussy infant may be soothed by using a pacifier. If you are unable to soothe an irritable infant, you may need to wait until he or she falls asleep. For older children, you can allow them to apply their own arm and leg electrodes. Adolescents may prefer to be alone with you during the procedure. Ask them if they would like their parent(s) to stay or leave.

When the ECG tracing is completed, talk about the procedure. Give verbal praise and be supportive. Reward the child, if appropriate for the age. Give stickers or a special trip to the playroom.

Smaller electrodes should be used for pediatric patients. Special smaller electrodes are available. Depending on the size of the child, you may need to trim adult electrodes. In addition, frequently you will need to adjust the paper speed to 50mm/sec for infants or children with very fast heart rates. This will allow the physician to view each of the deflections on the ECG tracing. If you make this adjustment, be sure to note it on the ECG recording when completed.

Figure 4-13: For infants and small children, you may need to place V3 on the right side of the chest to prevent crowding of the chest electrodes. This alternate method of placement is known as V3R and is sometimes used on adults.

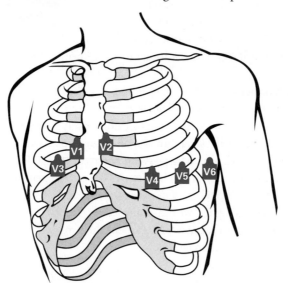

An ECG for a child is performed with the same lead placement as for an adult. The chest lead V6 must be placed exactly in the midaxillary line. Because of the small size of the chest, correct placement becomes even more important. Small differences in placement can make a difference in the ECG tracing. Because of crowding on the chest, it may be necessary to move the V3 lead to the right side of the chest. It should be placed on the right side in the same location as it normally would be on the left. This is known as a V3 right (V3R) (see Figure 4-13).

Special Patient Considerations

Occasionally you will need to record lead tracings other than the basic 12. You may need to record a heart rhythm strip, which is a single strip showing only one lead tracing. The heart rhythm is usually produced in lead II and is about 10 seconds of running time. Many of the newer ECG machines will print this strip on the bottom of the 12-lead tracing or following the completion of the 12-lead recording. A rhythm strip will be used to check for heart rhythm abnormalities. You may also be asked to provide a V3R on an adult.

You may encounter other circumstances that require you to make modifications to the basic 12-lead procedure. When changes in the placement of leads is necessary for any reason, a note should be included on the tracing. Consider the following when placing leads and recording tracings in a patient's chart:

- Do not place the electrode on a woman's breast. Lift the breast and place the electrode under it. If this is done, note on the ECG tracing that the electrodes are placed lower than required.

- If a woman has had a mastectomy, note this on the ECG tracing. It may alter the ECG results.

- If the patient is an amputee, place the limb leads on the upper chest and lower abdomen instead of the arms and legs. Make sure the leads are in the same place on each side of the body.

- A pregnant woman should have the lower limb leads placed on the thighs, not the abdomen. Place the patient on her left side slightly, by using a small rolled towel under the right hip. Document on the ECG that the patient is pregnant and the number of months.

- Geriatric patients generally have thin skin, which is part of the normal aging process. Apply the electrodes carefully and remove gently to prevent damage to their skin. Geriatric patients may have some readings on the ECG tracing that are age-related and are considered normal.

- If the patient is unable to lie on his or her back, be sure to indicate on the tracing the position of the patient during the tracing.

- When someone is in a permanent fetal position with their arms drawn tightly over their chest, you may need to place the electrodes on the back. They will need to be positioned over the heart on the left side of the back. Today's small, thin, disposable electrodes are easier to place under a patient's arms, so place on the back only if necessary.

- A condition that would require the changing of lead placement is **dextrocardia,** when the left ventricle, left atrium, aortic arch, and stomach are located on the right side of the chest. The leads should be reversed (mirror image) from the usual lead placement. This is the only case where the aVR tracing will produce a positive deflection. On the ECG tracing report, you should indicate that you did a right-side ECG (see Figure 4-14).

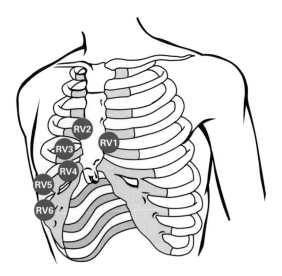

Figure 4-14: Use these lead placements for patients with dextrocardia, a condition in which the left ventricle, left atrium, aortic arch, and stomach are located on the right side of the chest.

Handling Emergencies

Code blue

During a code blue emergency, be ready to perform the tracing as quickly and efficiently as possible. An ECG is usually ordered "stat" in these situations. Enter the patient's information into the ECG machine and remain available but out of the way until the ECG is needed. You may need to take just the machine into the room and not the cart, if space is limited.

Because the patient's condition changes frequently during a code blue emergency, you may need to perform two ECGs in a row. Perform the first ECG and leave the electrodes in place in order to perform the second ECG quickly. Indicate on the tracing "repeat ECG—same lead placement." This will make the physician aware that the electrodes were not removed in between tracings.

Seizure

If a patient has a **seizure** during the ECG, stay with him or her. Protect the patient from injury. Do not try to restrain the patient. Call for help and report the seizure. Once the seizure is over, perform the ECG again and write on the ECG strip "postseizure."

Table 5-1 Calculating heart rates with a regular rhythm

Small boxes in P-P or R-R interval	Heart rate	Small boxes in P-P or R-R interval	Heart rate	Small boxes in P-P or R-R interval	Heart rate
4	375	20	75	36	42
5	300	21	71	37	40
6	250	22	68	38	39
7	214	23	65	39	38
8	188	24	62	40	38
9	167	25	60	41	37
10	150	26	58	42	36
11	136	27	55	43	35
12	125	28	54	44	34
13	115	29	52	45	33
14	107	30	50	46	33
15	100	31	48	47	32
16	94	32	47	48	31
17	88	33	45	49	31
18	83	34	44	50	30
19	79	35	43		

is often used in emergencies to determine an estimated heart rate (pulse rate) for the patient.

Step 3: Identifying the P wave configuration

Analyzing P waves and their relationship with the QRS complex is necessary to determine the type of dysrhythmia. The P wave reflects the atrial contraction and how the electrical current is moving through the atria. The relationship between the P wave and QRS complex provides information regarding the coordination between atrial and ventricular contractions. Several questions need to be answered when analyzing the P wave.

- *Are the shapes and waveforms all the same?* If they appear to be different, the route in which the current is moving through the atria is not on the same pathway. Sometimes the P wave may not exist.
- *Does each P wave have a QRS complex following it?* In normal conduction pathways, the QRS complex always follows the P wave. If there are additional P waves or QRS complexes present without a P wave in front, the normal conduction pathway may not have been used and the atria and ventricles are not contracting together.

Step 4: Measuring the PR interval

The PR interval measures the length of time it takes the electrical current to be initiated at the SA node and travel through the electrical current pathway to cause a ventricular contraction. The PR interval is determined by measuring from the beginning

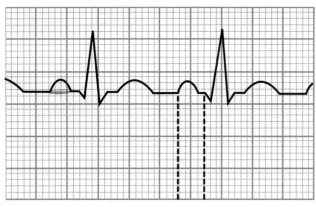

Figure 5-4: Measuring the PR interval

of the P wave, or its up slope, to the beginning of the QRS complex. (Please review Figure 2-10 on page 26, if necessary.) The normal range of the PR interval is .12 to .20 seconds (see Figure 5-4).

When determining the measurements, the time interval should always be in multiples of .02 seconds, which represents one-half of the smallest box. To effectively determine measurements to .01 second, the small box on the ECG paper would need to be divided into four smaller divisions. This can be done effectively only with a computer, not a practitioner's eyes.

PR intervals are also evaluated to ensure that the measurements are the same from one PR interval to the next. If the intervals have different measurements, either the electrical current is being delayed for some reason or it may be initiating from locations other than the SA node.

Step 5: Measuring the QRS duration

Measuring the QRS complex is essential in determining the duration of time it takes for the ventricles to depolarize or contract. This information is helpful in discriminating between different dysrhythmias. If the QRS complex is narrow, or within the normal limits of .06 to .10 seconds, current has traveled through the normal ventricular conduction pathways to activate the ventricles to contract. When the QRS complex is wide, or greater than .12 seconds, the current is taking longer than normal to contract the ventricles.

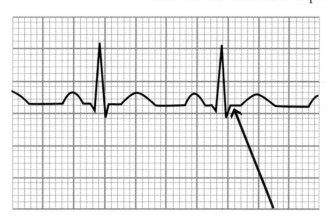

Figure 5-5: Locating the J point

To measure the QRS complex, place the first caliper point where the QRS complex starts and the second point at the **J point** (see Figure 5-5). The J point is located where the S wave stops and the ST segment is initiated. It marks the point at which depolarization is completed and repolarization begins. It is important to carefully identify this ending point of the QRS complex, since many times the ST segment may not be at the isoelectric line.

Several questions need to be answered when determining the QRS measurement (see Figure 5-6).

• Are all the QRS complexes of equal length?

• What is the actual measurement, and is it within the normal limits?

• Do all QRS complexes look alike, and are the unusual QRS complexes associated with an ectopic beat?

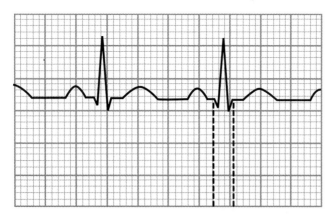

Figure 5-6: Measuring the QRS duration

After you have completed these five steps of identifying the components of the rhythm, you will then compare the information to the specific criteria for classifying each of the dysrhythmias. The rest of this chapter explains the specific criteria for classification related to common rhythms and dysrhythmias that will help you identify the various ECG rhythms.

Rhythms Originating from the Sinus Node (Sinus Beat)

The sinoatrial (SA) node or normal pacemaker generates an electrical impulse that travels through the normal conduction pathway to cause the myocardium to depolarize. Electrical current starts at the SA node and travels the normal conduction pathway to the AV node and continues through the Bundle of His and bundle branches to the ventricles. Because the rhythm starts at the SA node it is called sinus rhythm. The electrical current is produced at the sinus node at a rate of 60 to 100 beats per minute. The rates of the rhythm will vary, and the types of sinus beats may include sinus rhythm, sinus bradycardia, sinus tachycardia, and sinus arrhythmia.

Sinus rhythm

Sinus rhythm (SR) is reflective of a normally functioning conduction system. The electrical current is following the normal conduction pathway without interference from other bodily systems or disease processes (see Figure 5-7).

Criteria for classification

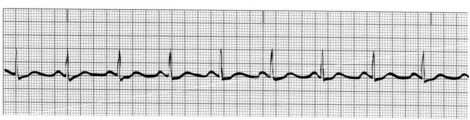

Figure 5-7: Sinus rhythm

- *Rhythm:* The intervals between the two P and two R waves will occur in a consistent pattern.
- *Rate:* Both the atrial and ventricular rate will be between 60 and 100 beats.
- *P wave configuration:* The P waves will have the same shape and are usually upright in deflection on the rhythm strip. A P wave will appear in front of every QRS complex.
- *PR interval:* The PR interval measurement will be between .12 and .20 seconds, which is within normal limits. Each PR interval will be the same, without any variations.
- *QRS duration:* The QRS duration measurement will be between .06 and .10 seconds, which is within normal limits. Each QRS duration will be without any variations from PQRST complex to complex.

TROUBLESHOOTING

The patient you are monitoring is very pale and appears to be breathing very fast. Even though the patient's rhythm is SR, you should report it to the licensed practitioner immediately because the patient is showing two signs of decreased cardiac output: pale skin and respiratory difficulty.

Table 5-2 Signs and symptoms of decreased cardiac output

Observe for any of these signs and symptoms associated with decreased cardiac output when administering an ECG.

Neurological	Cardiac	Respiratory	Urinary	Peripheral
■ Change in mental status ■ Light-headedness ■ Dizziness ■ Confusion ■ Loss of consciousness	■ Chest pain ■ Palpitation ■ Chest discomfort ■ Enlarged cardiac size ■ Congestive heart failure	■ Difficulty breathing ■ Shortness of breath ■ Frothy sputum ■ Fluid present in lungs ■ Lung congestion	■ Decreased urinary output of less than 30 cc in one hour	■ Hypotension ■ Pale skin ■ Skin cool and clammy to the touch

How the patient is affected and what you should know

Sinus rhythm is the desired rhythm. Patients with this rhythm should have normal cardiac output. Normal cardiac output means that the heart is beating adequately, pumping blood to the body's organs to maintain normal function. Signs and symptoms of adequate cardiac output include an alert and oriented patient with no difficulty breathing, no chest pain or pressure, and a stable blood pressure.

Because this is a normal rhythm, no intervention is necessary. If the patient's rhythm returns to sinus rhythm from another dysrhythmia, it is always important to make sure that the patient is not experiencing problems with low cardiac output, which indicates that the heart is not pumping adequately (see Table 5-2). Any time a patient displays symptoms of low cardiac output, a licensed practitioner needs to be informed for further assessment.

LAW AND ETHICS - The ECG rhythm, which is considered a legal document, needs to be included in the patient's medical record. The patient's name and the date and time must be identified on each rhythm strip. Documentation of the ECG rhythm and the patient's response helps support the reason for the medical treatment.

Sinus bradycardia

Sinus bradycardia (SB) is a rhythm of less than 60 beats per minute (see Figure 5-8). SB originates from the SA node and travels the normal conduction pathway. The only difference between this rhythm and SR is that the rate is less than the normal inherent rate of the SA node.

Criteria for classification

- *Rhythm:* The R-R interval and P-P interval will occur on a regular and constant basis.
- *Rate:* The atrial and ventricular rates will be equal and between 40 and 60 beats per minute.
- *P wave configuration:* The shapes of each of the P waves are identical. There is a P wave in front of each of the QRS complexes. No additional P waves or QRS complexes are noted.

Figure 5-8: Sinus bradycardia

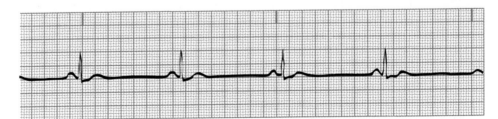

- **PR interval:** The PR interval measurement will be between .12 and .20 seconds, which is within normal limits. Each PR interval will be the same.
- **QRS duration:** The QRS duration measurement will be between .06 and .10 seconds, which is within normal limits. Each QRS duration will be the same, without any variations from QRS complex to complex.

How the patient is affected and what you should know

The patient who exhibits SB may or may not experience signs and symptoms of low cardiac output. When administering an ECG to a patient with a slow heart rate, it is important to observe for the symptoms of low cardiac output (see Table 5-2). Remember, though the patient may look all right, he or she can quickly experience difficulties with low cardiac output. When you observe symptoms of low cardiac output, report any findings to a licensed practitioner immediately. This rhythm may require drug administration or application of a pacemaker.

Sinus tachycardia

Sinus tachycardia (ST) is a condition in which the SA node fires and the electrical impulse travels through the normal conduction pathway but the rate of impulse firing is faster than 100 beats per minute (see Figure 5-9).

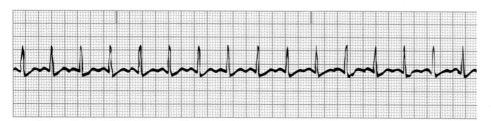

Figure 5-9: Sinus tachycardia

Criteria for classification

- **Rhythm:** The R-R interval and P-P interval will be equal and constant.
- **Rate:** Both the atrial and ventricular rates will be the same, between 100 and 150 beats per minute.
- **P wave configuration:** The P waves will have the same shape and usually are upright in deflection on the rhythm strip. There will be a P wave in front of every QRS complex.
- **PR interval:** The PR interval measurement will be between .12 and .20 seconds. This is within normal limits. Each PR interval will be the same, without any variations.
- **QRS duration:** The QRS duration measurement will be between .06 and .10 seconds, which is within normal limits. Each QRS duration will be the same, without any variations from QRS complex to complex.

How the patient is affected and what you should know

The effect of this rhythm on the patient depends on the rate of tachycardia above the patient's normal resting heart rate. For example, if the patient's normal resting heart rate is 90 and now the patient is exhibiting a rate of 108 beats per minute after walking the hallway, the tachycardia would be expected and is viewed as the patient's normal response to exercise. However, if the patient's normal heart rate is 60 and it is now 140, the patient is probably experiencing symptoms of low cardiac output. Often the patient will complain of **palpitations** or "heart fluttering" with faster rates. If the patient has had a recent myocardial infarction, ST is considered to be more serious or even life threatening.

When caring for a patient who is experiencing ST, first observe for signs and symptoms of low cardiac output. If evidence of low cardiac output is observed, a licensed practitioner should be notified immediately. Medication may need to be administered by a licensed practitioner.

Sinus arrhythmia

Sinus arrhythmia (SA) is a condition in which the heart rate remains within normal limits but is influenced by the respiratory cycle and variations of **vagal tone** (a condition in which impulses over the vagus nerve cause a decrease in heart rate), causing the rhythm to be irregular. For instance, when a patient inhales air, the pressure inside the chest cavity increases, causing pressure on the heart, specifically the sinoatrial node. The heart rate will slow with this increase in pressure. As the patient exhales, the chest cavity pressure decreases, allowing the SA node to fire more easily. Therefore, the heart rate will increase during exhalation (see Figure 5-10).

Figure 5-10: Sinus arrhythmia

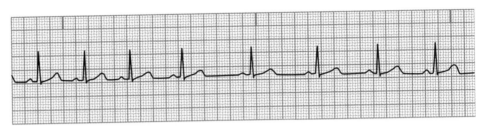

Criteria for classification

- *Rhythm:* The interval between the P-P and R-R waves will occur at irregular periods.
- *Rate:* Both the atrial and ventricular rates will be the same, between 60 and 100 beats per minute.
- *P wave configuration:* The P waves will have the same shape and usually are upright in deflection on the rhythm strip. There will be a P wave in front of every QRS complex.
- *PR interval:* The PR interval measurement will be between .12 and .20 seconds. Each PR interval will be the same, without any variations.
- *QRS duration:* The QRS duration measurement will be between .06 and .10 seconds. Each QRS duration will be the same, without any variations from QRS complex to complex.

How the patient is affected and what you should know

Patients usually show no clinical signs or symptoms with sinus arrhythmia. If the irregularity is severe enough to decrease the heart rate to the 40s, the patient may complain of palpitations or dizziness. This depends on how slow the heart beats when the SA node is suppressed from the respiratory or vagal influences. You should notify the physician or other licensed practitioner when the heart rate slows below 50 or the patient complains of dizziness or palpitations. A copy of the rhythm strip should be mounted on the patient's medical record for documentation.

Sinus arrest

Sinus arrest occurs when the SA node stops firing, causing a pause in electrical activity. During the pause, no electrical impulse is initiated or sent through the normal conduction system to cause either an atrial or a ventricular contraction (see Figure 5-11).

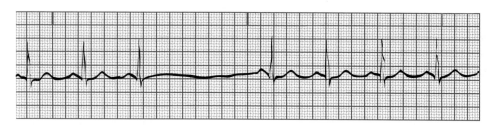

Figure 5-11: Sinus arrest

Criteria for classification

- *Rhythm:* The interval between the P-P and R-R waves will occur at irregular periods.
- *Rate:* Both the atrial and ventricular rates will be the same. The rate will vary depending on the amount of electrical activity occurring from the SA node.
- *P wave configuration:* The P waves will have the same shape and usually are upright in deflection on the rhythm strip. There will be a P wave in front of every QRS complex.
- *PR interval:* The PR interval measurement will be between .12 and .20 seconds, which is within normal limits. Each PR interval will be the same, without any variations.
- *QRS duration:* The QRS duration measurement will be between .06 and .10 seconds, which is within normal limits. Each QRS duration will be the same, without any variations from QRS complex to complex.
- *Length of pause:* The length of pause needs to be measured to determine how long the heart had no rhythm. To measure, place the calipers on the R-R interval around the pause. Once the time frame is determined, calculate the length of time for the pause by multiplying the number of boxes by .04 seconds. The frequency of pauses is also noted because the more frequent the pauses, the more urgent the situation.

How the patient is affected and what you should know

The seriousness of sinus arrest depends on the length of the pause. The patient will experience signs and symptoms of decreased cardiac output if the pause is two seconds long and occurs on a frequent basis. The pauses may also cause periods of **ischemia** (when cells are deprived of oxygen), hypotension, dizziness, and **syncope** (loss of consciousness).

The patient may initially appear to be asymptomatic (without symptoms) and then develop signs and symptoms of low cardiac output. Therefore, it is important to observe the patient frequently for signs of low cardiac output. Notify a licensed practitioner of these symptoms and provide information about the frequency and length of pauses. The patient will require immediate treatment.

Rhythms Originating From the Atria

Atrial dysrhythmia is caused by an ectopic beat in either the right or the left atria. However, the atrial origin is outside the SA node, which interrupts the inherent rate

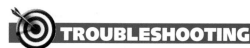

TROUBLESHOOTING

If the sinus arrest lasts longer than 6 seconds, this rhythm is considered **asystole,** indicating that no electrical current is traveling through the cardiac conduction system. Asystole is considered a life-threatening dysrhythmia that requires immediate CPR and code blue measures.

of the SA node. The heart works on the principle that the fastest impulse will control the heart rate. Since the atrial ectopic beat is generating electrical impulses faster than the SA node, the ectopic beat will override the SA node impulse and cause the atria and ventricles to depolarize. Dysrhythmias that are caused by the atrial ectopic site include premature atrial contraction, atrial tachycardia, atrial flutter, and atrial fibrillation.

Atrial dysrhythmias occur from conditions that cause pressure on the atria such as damage to the atria from myocardial infarction, valvular problems, or **neurological** influences (pertaining to the nervous system). When the area is stressed or damaged, the cells become unstable, and the electrical state may cause depolarization to occur more easily.

Premature atrial contraction

Premature atrial contractions (PACs) are electrical impulses that originate in the atria and initiate an early impulse that interrupts the inherent regular rhythm (see Figure 5-12).

Figure 5-12: Premature atrial contraction

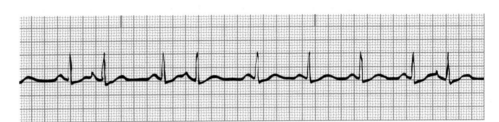

Criteria for classification

- **Rhythm:** The regularity between the P-P interval and R-R interval is constant with the exception of the early complexes. There will be a section of the rhythm that is regular and occasionally an early complex.
- **Rate:** The rates of the atria and ventricles will usually be within normal limits of 60 to 100, depending on the frequency of the PACs.
- **P wave configuration:** The P waves will have the same configuration and shape. The early beat will have a different shape than the rest of the P waves on the strip. This P wave may be flattened, notched, **biphasic** (have two phases), or otherwise unusual. It may even be hidden within the T wave of the preceding complex. Evidence that the P wave is hidden within the T wave includes a notch in the T wave, a pointed shape, or being taller than the other T waves.
- **PR interval:** The PR interval will measure within normal limits of .12 to .20 seconds. The early beat will probably have a different PR measurement than the normal complexes but will be within normal limits.
- **QRS duration:** The QRS duration will be within normal limits of .06 to .10 seconds.

Determine the underlying rhythm of SR, SB, ST, or SA when identifying PACs. The rhythm strip must be labeled with this underlying rhythm and the type of PAC. An example of this terminology is "sinus rhythm with trigeminal PACs" (**trigeminy** refers to a pattern in which every third complex is a premature beat).

How the patient is affected and what you should know

With each PAC, the atria do not achieve the maximum blood capacity prior to contraction. This lack of blood causes a decrease in cardiac output and less volume in the ventricles prior to ventricular contraction. Therefore, in the patient who has prior cardiac disease, frequent PACs can cause the patient to experience symptoms of low cardiac output.

When caring for a patient with PACs, observe the patient for signs and symptoms of low cardiac output. Monitoring the amount or frequency of PACs is essential. The patient may complain of palpitations from the early beats. The severity of the patient's complaints is related to the frequency of the PACs. In addition, frequent PACs may indicate that a more serious atrial dysrhythmia may follow. The more frequent occurrence indicates that the ectopic **focus** (cardiac cell that functions as an ectopic beat) may continue and take control of the heart rate. Any observation of low cardiac output should be communicated to a licensed practitioner for appropriate treatment.

Atrial flutter

Atrial flutter (A flutter) occurs when a rapid impulse originates in the atrial tissue. The ectopic focus may be originating from ischemic areas of the heart with enhanced **automaticity** (ability to initiate an electrical current) or from a reentry pathway. A reentry pathway is an extra pathway that has developed where a group of cells will generate an impulse faster than the SA node. This impulse then follows a route that allows the impulse to reach the AV node quicker than the normal conduction pathway. The reentry pathway is similar to finding a short cut to work or school to bypass the normal traffic route to get you to your destination faster. The electrical current or rhythm is recorded in a characteristic saw-tooth pattern (see Figure 5-13). This atrial activity is called flutter waves. Most often this is a transient dysrhythmia that will lead to more serious atrial dysrhythmia if not treated.

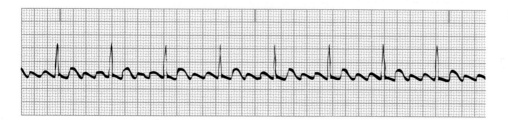

Figure 5-13: Atrial flutter

Criteria for classification

- **Rhythm:** The P-P interval or flutter-to-flutter waves will be regular. The interval set with the calipers will stay constant throughout the rhythm. The R-R interval is usually irregular, but occasionally it may be regular in pattern. The regularity of the R-R interval will depend on the ability of the AV node to limit impulses to ventricles.

- **Rate:** The atrial rate will be between 250 and 350 beats per minute.

- **P wave configuration:** P waves are not seen, and only flutter waves are present. These flutter waves resemble a "saw-tooth" or "picket fence." They will be seen best in leads II, III, and aVF. The correlation between P waves and QRS complexes no longer exists. There will be more flutter waves than QRS complexes.

- **PR interval:** No identifiable P wave exists, so the PR interval cannot be measured.

- **QRS duration:** The QRS duration will be within normal limits of .06 seconds to .10 seconds.

How the patient is affected and what you should know

The **atrial kick,** which occurs when blood is ejected into the ventricles by the atria immediately prior to ventricular systole, is no longer present since the atria do not contract completely, followed by a delay in the ventricular contraction. This loss in atrial kick contributes to a 10% to 30% decrease in cardiac output. Some patients may tolerate this if the heart rate is within normal limits of 60 to 100 beats per minute. But once the heart rate increases significantly and loss of the atrial kick occurs, the patient will demonstrate signs and symptoms of low cardiac output.

When atrial flutter occurs, notify the licensed practitioner to implement a treatment plan, which usually includes oxygen therapy to ensure adequate supply to the vital organs. The patient is monitored continuously to determine if the rhythm converts to a sinus rhythm or progresses to atrial fibrillation. A continuous rhythm strip is needed to document if any changes occurred as a result of the medical intervention. Always indicate on the rhythm strip the type of intervention that is being implemented. The ECG strips are then mounted and saved in the patient's medical record or chart.

Atrial fibrillation

Atrial fibrillation (A fib.) occurs when electrical impulses come from areas of reentry pathways or multiple ectopic foci. Each electrical impulse results in depolarization of only a small group of atrial cells rather than the whole atria. This results in the atria not contracting as a whole, causing it to quiver, similar to a bowl of Jell-O™ when shaken. Multiple atrial activity is recorded as a chaotic wave, often with the appearance of fine scribbles (see Figure 5-14). No P wave can be identified. The waveform of the chaotic "scribbles" is referred to as fibrillatory waves or f waves.

Figure 5-14: Atrial fibrillation

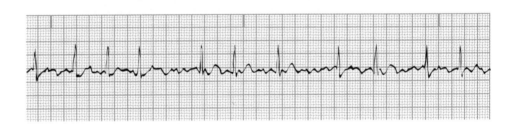

Criteria for classification

- ***Rhythm:*** The P-P interval is unable to be determined because of the fibrillatory waves or f waves. The R-R interval is irregular.

- ***Rate:*** Atrial rate, if measurable, will be from 375 to 700 beats per minute. It is difficult to determine the atrial rates because each fibrillatory wave is not easy to identify or measure. The ventricular rate is initially between 160 and 180 beats per minute prior to administering medication. Once medication is provided, the ventricular rate is considered under control if the rate is between 60 and 100 beats per minute.

- ***P wave configuration:*** The P waves cannot be identified. There is chaotic electrical activity, or f waves may be seen.

- ***PR interval:*** The PR interval cannot be measured, since the P wave is not identifiable.

- ***QRS duration:*** The QRS duration will be within normal limits of .06 to .10 seconds and irregular.

How the patient is affected and what you should know

The patient will exhibit signs and symptoms of decreased cardiac output. The patient usually has limited cardiac function because of pre-existing cardiac conditions, so with the loss of atrial kick, the patient's cardiac output will decrease significantly. Once the heart rate is controlled within the range of 60 to 100 beats per minute, the patient may be able to tolerate the loss of the atrial kick.

Blood will begin to collect in the atria because they are not contracting completely, allowing the opportunity for a clot or thrombus to form. Therefore, the patient has an increased risk of developing and sending an embolism (traveling blood clot) out into the body's systemic circulation, which can then migrate to other vital organs, such as the lungs or brain. The patient may develop a cerebral vascular accident (CVA), myocardial infarction (MI), pulmonary embolism, renal infarction, or an embolism in any place that the arterial blood is transported. Essentially, the heart is playing Russian roulette with us because there is no way to predict where the embolism will travel in the body to cause serious damage or even sudden death.

Patients who exhibit atrial fibrillation must be observed for low cardiac output. The rhythm needs to be monitored closely as the medication or electrical cardioversion (defibrillation) is attempted. Report any complications or vital sign changes to the licensed practitioner immediately.

Rhythms Originating from the Atrial-Junction Node

The AV (atrial-ventricular) node is sometimes referred to as the AV junction. Though abnormal, these AV node cells, which possess the property of automaticity, can function as a pacemaker. The inherent rate of the AV node is between 40 and 60 beats per minute. When the AV node instead of the SA node initiates the electrical impulse, the rhythm is referred to as a junctional dysrhythmia. With junctional rhythms, it is important to understand that the electrical current is initiated from the AV junction. Junctional rhythms are suggestive of more serious conditions with the electrical conduction system in the heart. The AV node is the backup pacemaker for the heart after the SA node. Junctional rhythm, accelerated junctional rhythm, and junctional tachycardia are all conditions in which the SA node has been injured and the AV node functions as the pacemaker of the heart.

Junctional rhythm

Junctional rhythm (JR) originates at AV junctional tissue, producing retrograde (backwards) depolarization of atrial tissue, and at the same time, stimulates the depolarization of ventricles (see Figure 5-15).

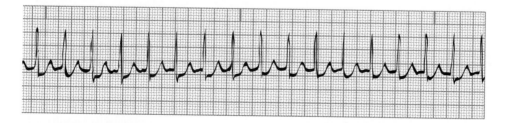

Figure 5-15: Junctional rhythm

Criteria for classification

- **Rhythm:** The P-P and R-R intervals are regular and at similar intervals. The P-P interval may be difficult to measure due to the location of the P wave.

- **Rate:** If the P wave is identifiable, the rate will be 40 to 60 beats per minute. The ventricular rate will be 40 to 60 beats per minute.
- **P wave configuration:** The P wave is usually inverted and may precede, follow, or fall within the QRS complex. It may not be visible at all on the rhythm strip.
- **PR interval:** If the P wave is before the QRS complex, the PR interval will measure less than .12 seconds and will be constant. If the P wave is not before the QRS complex, the PR interval cannot be determined.
- **QRS duration:** The QRS duration will be within normal limits of .06 to .10 seconds.

How the patient is affected and what you should know

The patient has a slower heart rate than normal and loses the atrial kick due to the shortening of the interval between the atrial depolarization and ventricular depolarization. These conditions cause the patient to exhibit symptoms of low cardiac output. Common signs and symptoms of low cardiac output displayed include **hypotension** (low blood pressure) and altered mental status such as confusion or disorientation. Observe for symptoms and monitor the ECG tracing in case a more serious dysrhythmia occurs. Report the presence of JR and your observations of the patient to a licensed practitioner for appropriate medical treatment.

Supraventricular Dysrhythmias

A supraventricular tachycardia (SVT) is a classification of rapid heartbeats, usually occurring at a rate greater than 150 beats per minute (see Figure 5-16). **Supraventricular** refers to an ectopic focus originating above the ventricles, in the atria, or junctional region of the heart. The heart is beating so fast that it is difficult to determine if the source of origin is from the sinus node, atria, or the AV junction. Because the heart rate is so rapid, the atria are contracting as soon as the ventricles are relaxing. This causes the P waves (atrial contraction) to become difficult to identify, because they may occur at the same time as the T waves (ventricle relaxation). Rhythms that fall into this category are identified in Table 5-3.

The primary difficulty in classifying the actual rhythm is identifying where the tachycardia originates. The P wave may appear before, after, or during the QRS complex, depending on the origin. The PR interval measurement is difficult to assess since you cannot often see the initial up swing of the P wave.

Figure 5-16:
Supraventricular tachycardia

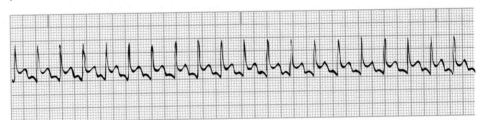

Table 5-3 Dysrhythmias associated with supraventricular tachycardia		
Sinus Node	**Atrium**	**Junctional**
Sinus tachycardia	Atrial tachycardia	Junctional tachycardia
	Atrial flutter	
	Atrial fibrillation	

Criteria for classification

- **Rhythm:** The ventricular (R-R) rhythm is usually regular or with minimal irregularity from R-R interval. The atrial rhythm may or may not be seen. This is because other electrical activity is occurring at the same time. Remember, the ECG will record only the activity it "sees" in each lead. The atrial activity is small compared to ventricular activity; therefore, the ventricular activity is the largest amount of energy seen when the ECG tracing is recorded. Depending on whether the P waves are seen, you may not be able to determine regular P waves. If identifiable, they are usually regular.

- **Rate:** The ventricular rate is 150 to 350 beats per minute. The atrial rate will be difficult to determine when P waves are unidentifiable.

- **P wave configuration:** The P waves are usually not identified when the heart rate is this rapid. Remember that when the heart rate increases, the time interval between atrial contraction and ventricular relaxation decreases. Therefore, if there is a P wave present, it may occur simultaneously with the T wave and may be buried within it. The P wave may occur before, during, or after the QRS complex.

- **PR interval:** Usually the PR interval is unable to be determined because the beginning of the P wave cannot be clearly identified.

- **QRS duration:** The QRS measurement is considered within normal limits when measured at .06 to .10 seconds.

How the patient is affected and what you should know

There are various supraventricular dysrhythmias, all of which may cause the patient to exhibit the same signs and symptoms. The patient may be in either a stable or an unstable condition. The stable patient (one without signs and symptoms of decreased cardiac output) may only complain of palpitations and state, "I'm just not feeling right" or "My heart is fluttering." When the patient's condition is *unstable*, he or she may experience any symptom of low cardiac output, which is reflective of the heart not pumping effectively to other body systems. Many patients may present initially with a stable condition, and then a few minutes later experience unstable symptoms such as those presented in Table 5-2 on page 80.

Observe the patient for symptoms of low cardiac output; symptoms and rhythm changes need to be communicated quickly to a licensed practitioner for appropriate medical treatment. Because tachycardia severely deprives the heart of oxygen, treatment should begin as early as possible. It is difficult to predict how long a patient's heart can beat at a rapid rate before it begins to affect the other body systems.

> **LAW AND ETHICS** - Your role regarding evaluation of the rhythm strip and assessment of the patient will depend on your training and place of employment. Working outside of your scope of practice is illegal, and you could be held liable for performing tasks that are not part of your role as a health care professional.

Heart Block Rhythms

In heart block rhythms, the electrical current has difficulty traveling along the normal conduction pathway, causing a delay in or absence of ventricular depolarization. The degree of blockage is dependent on the area affected and the cause of the delay or blockage. There are three levels of heart blocks.

First degree AV block

First degree AV block is a *delay* in electrical conduction from the SA node to the AV node, usually around the AV node, which prevents an electrical impulse from traveling to the ventricular conduction system (see Figure 5-17). The condition is similar to being in a traffic jam. You still arrive at your destination, but it takes you longer to get there. Electrical current from the SA node will still stimulate ventricular depolarization, but the time it takes to arrive in the ventricles is longer than normal.

Figure 5-17: First degree AV block

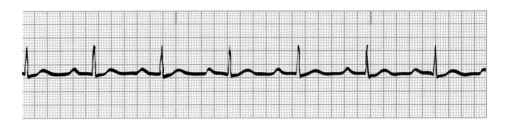

Criteria for classification

- *Rhythm:* The regularity between the P-P interval and the R-R interval is constant.

- *Rate:* The rate of the atria and ventricles will usually be within normal limits of 60 to 100 beats per minute.

- *P wave configuration:* The P waves will have the same configuration and shape. Each QRS complex will have a P wave before it. There will be the same number of P waves as QRS complexes.

- *PR interval:* The PR interval will be greater than .20 seconds.

- *QRS duration:* The QRS duration will be within normal limits of .06 to .10 seconds.

How the patient is affected and what you should know

The patient will be able to maintain normal cardiac output. No change in the patient should occur with this rhythm. Monitor and observe for further degeneration and development of other heart blocks and report if they occur. It is important to observe the **cardiac output parameters**—to assess the blood supply to the vital organs—and to determine how well the patient is tolerating the dysrhythmia.

Second degree AV block, Mobitz I (Wenckebach)

Second degree heart block has some **blocked or nonconducted** electrical **impulses** from the SA node to the ventricles at the AV junction region. These are impulses that occur too soon after the preceding impulsing, causing a period when no other impulses can occur in the ventricles. However, some electrical impulses are still being conducted along the normal conduction pathway. There are currently two different types of second degree heart blocks, which were first discovered by Dr. Mobitz. Dr. Wenckebach further investigated the rhythm and was able to identify a similar blockage pattern, but it was different from the one Dr. Mobitz observed. The rhythm Dr. Wenckebach observed was specifically labeled second degree AV block, Mobitz I, although it is often referred to as a Wenckebach rhythm. It is caused when diseased or injured AV node tissue conducts the electrical impulse to the ventricular conduction pathway with increasing difficulty, causing a delay in time until one of the atrial impulses fails to be conducted or is blocked. After the dropped atrial impulse, the AV node resets itself to be able to handle future impulses more quickly and then progressively gets more difficult until it drops or is blocked again. This pattern will repeat itself (see Figure 5-18).

Step 5. *Is AV delay appropriate?* (For AV sequential pacemakers only)
Measuring from the atrial spike to the ventricular spike, or from the beginning of the P wave to the ventricular spike, will give you the AV delay interval. This time frame should be the same as the AV delay set on the pacemaker program. This information should be available on the patient's medical record or pacemaker information card.

Step 6. *Is ventricular sensing appropriate?*
The ECG tracing needs to be evaluated for the presence of ventricular spikes with the wide QRS complex following the spike. Occasionally the patient's own conduction system will work appropriately, as evidenced by a normal P wave and/or QRS complex. If the ventricular contraction occurred normally before the time interval of when the pacemaker would send a ventricular impulse, the pacemaker generator will be **inhibited,** or stopped. This is evidenced by the absence of a ventricular spike.

Step 7. *Is ventricular capture present?*
Every ventricular spike should have a wide QRS complex after it to indicate that the electrical current caused the cells to depolarize. Appearance of the QRS complex after the spike indicates that ventricular capture occurred.

Pacemaker complications relative to the ECG tracing

Pacemaker generators use lithium batteries to create an electrical impulse. As with any battery, the charge of the battery will decrease to the point where the battery needs to be replaced. If a pacemaker is losing its ability to function properly, this failure will be evident on the ECG tracings. These changes in rhythms are often referred to as complications of the pacemaker. Complications include slower firing rates than set, less effective sensing capabilities, and lower electrical current than predetermined.

Another pacemaker complication is related to the functioning of the pacemaker generator when the sensing capability is too low. If sensing capability is low, the pacemaker will not be able to "see" the normal contractions occurring in the sensing chamber. Therefore, electrical impulses will not be inhibited but may actually be **triggered,** sending an impulse to the myocardium because the normal electrical current of the heart's conduction system was not "seen."

There are several different reasons for pacemaker complications, but only four basic dysrhythmias are evident on the ECG tracing from these complications: **malfunctioning** (failure to pace), **malsensing** (failure to sense), **loss of capture** (failure to depolarize), and **oversensing** (perceiving electrical current from sources other than the heart) (see Table 5-6).

Responsibility in caring for patients with pacemakers requires recognizing normal pacemaker rhythms and possible complications. When you are performing an ECG or monitoring a patient with a pacemaker, you should be aware of the differences in the ECG waveforms, including the presences of a pacing spike, chamber depolarization characteristics, and an AV delay. If you observe complications of a pacemaker rhythm, immediately notify licensed personnel for appropriate treatment and interventions.

Table 5-6 Pacemaker complications

Complication	Cause	What Occurs	Patient Symptoms
Malfunctioning (failure to pace)	Pacemaker does not send electrical impulse to the myocardium	Pacemaker intervals are irregular and impulse is slower than set rate	Patient will most often experience hypotension, lightheadedness, and blackout periods due to bradycardia conditions
Malsensing (failure to sense)	Pacemaker does not sense the patient's own inherent rate	May send current to heart during relaxation (repolarization) phase; also known as **pacemaker competition** with the patient's own heart	With atrial pacing, atrial fibrillation can occur; with ventricular pacing, ventricular tachycardia or ventricular fibrillation can occur
Loss of capture (failure to depolarize)	Pacing activity occurs but myocardium is not depolarized	Pacing spikes will occur without capture waveform afterward	Symptoms depend on the basic dysrhythmia and the patient's condition prior to the pacemaker insertion
Oversensing	Pacemaker perceives electrical current from sources other than the heart	Either (1) the patient's own heart rate is recorded and is slower than the set rate of the pacemaker or (2) the pacemaker spikes and captures at a slower rate than set	Patient may have signs and symptoms of low cardiac output

Chapter Review

The Match Game: Match the following terms with their definitions. Place the appropriate letter on the line provided.

_____ 1. atrial kick

_____ 2. apnea

_____ 3. neurological

_____ 4. ischemia

_____ 5. vagal tone

_____ 6. syncope

_____ 7. inhibited

_____ 8. palpitations

_____ 9. supraventricular

_____ 10. J point

a. heartbeat sensation felt by the patient

b. electrical current is stopped from being sent to the myocardium

c. pertaining to the nervous system

d. patient loses consciousness

e. impulses on the vagal nerve cause inhibitory effect on the heart

f. an ectopic focus originating above the ventricles

g. point on the QRS complex at which depolarization is complete

h. absence of breathing

i. lack of oxygen to heart muscle cells

j. blood ejected into ventricles prior to ventricular systole

It's Your Choice: Circle the correct answer.

11. What is the rate of a normal sinus rhythm?

    a. 60 to 100 beats per minute

    b. 50 to 90 beats per minute

    c. 100 to 150 beats per minute

    d. 60 to 80 beats per minute

12. What sinus rhythm has a rate of less than 60 beats per minute?

    a. sinus tachycardia

    b. sinus bradycardia

    c. sinus arrythmia

    d. sinus rhythms

13. Which is *not* a question that needs to be answered when determining the QRS measurement?

    a. Are all the QRS complexes of equal length?

    b. What is the actual QRS measurement and is it within the normal limits?

    c. Do all QRS complexes look alike and are the unusual QRS complexes associated with an ectopic beat?

    d. Is the R-R pattern regular?

14. What sinus rhythm has a rate of more than 100 beats per minute?

    a. sinus tachycardia

    b. sinus bradycardia

    c. sinus arrhythmia

    d. sinus rhythms

15. What rhythm shows an irregularity during inspiration and expiration?

    a. sinus tachycardia

    b. sinus bradycardia

    c. sinus arrhythmia

    d. sinus rhythms

16. In which period of the cardiac cycle is a strong ventricular stimulus potentially dangerous?

    a. U wave

    b. P wave

    c. T wave

    d. QRS complex

17. The normal P-R interval is:

    a. .04 to .10 seconds

    b. .12 to .20 seconds

    c. .22 to .26 seconds

    d. .28 to .32 seconds

18. If a QRS complex is wider than 0.12 seconds, it most likely indicates

    a. normal ventricular conduction.

    b. delayed ventricular conduction.

    c. increased delay at the AV node.

    d. myocardial infarction.

19. What is the range of heart rate for ventricular fibrillation?

    a. 60 to 100 beats per minute

    b. 40 to 60 beats per minute

    c. 100 to 200 beats per minute

    d. >300 beats per minute

20. What is the normal, inherent rate for the AV junction?

    a. 60 to 100 beats per minute

    b. 40 to 60 beats per minute

    c. 100 to 160 beats per minute

    d. 20 to 40 beats per minute

21. Which of the following dysrhythmias is not considered part of the supraventricular tachycardia classification?

    a. atrial fibrillation

    b. sinus tachycardia

    c. ventricular tachycardia

    d. junctional tachycardia

22. What sign or symptom might a patient complain about when experiencing a supraventricular tachycardia in an unstable condition?

    a. back pain

    b. palpitations

    c. hypothyroidism

    d. chest pain and discomfort

23. The criterion needed to classify the dysrhythmia as a supraventricular tachycardia is

    a. a heart rate between 150 and 350 beats per minute.

    b. a wide QRS complex.

    c. a clear, easily identifiable P wave with the entire wave visualized.

    d. atrial and ventricular rates that are not the same.

24. What is the primary difficulty in determining a supraventricular rhythm?

    a. determining the ventricular rate

    b. determining the regularity

    c. measuring the QRS interval

    d. determining the origin of the tachycardia

25. When is the identification of the specific dysrhythmia important in terms of treatment of the patient?

    a. when the patient first complains of any signs or symptoms

    b. when the patient's heart rate has decreased to a rate of 100 to150 beats per minute

    c. during the treatment of a fast tachycardia situation

    d. after the rhythm has been converted to a normal rhythm and/or the heart rate is between 60 and 100 beats per minute

26. You observe a wide QRS complex while continuously monitoring a patient in lead II. Which lead placement is necessary to evaluate the location of blockage in the bundle branch system?

    a. lead I   **c.** lead III

    b. lead V4   **d.** lead V1

27. The labeling of the ECG rhythm strip for documentation of the bundle branch block should include what other information besides which bundle is being blocked?

 a. symptoms the patient is experiencing

 b. blood pressure reading

 c. presence of an MI diagnosis

 d. patient's inherent rhythm pattern

28. What is the minimum QRS measurement for a ventricular complex?

 a. .06 to .10 seconds

 b. .04 to .08 seconds

 c. less than .12 seconds

 d. greater than .12 seconds

29. What do you call two PVCs that are connected to each other without a normal beat in between?

 a. coupling or pair

 b. run of ventricular tachycardia

 c. frequent PVCs

 d. R-on-T PVCs

30. Which of the following is not one of the components to be evaluated on a pacemaker tracing?

 a. the presence of atrial and/or ventricular spikes

 b. the QT interval

 c. the characteristic patterns of the chambers captured after the spikes

 d. the AV delay period

The Match Game: Match the following terms related to electronic (artificial) pacemakers to their definitions.

_____ 31. pacemaker competition

_____ 32. pacemaker (electronic)

_____ 33. loss of capture

_____ 34. malsensing

_____ 35. malfunctioning

_____ 36. oversensing

_____ 37. triggered

_____ 38. capture

a. electrical current causes the myocardial tissue to depolarize (contract)

b. heart muscle responds to electrical stimulation and depolarizes (contracts)

c. device that delivers electrical energy to cause depolarization (contractions)

d. pacing activity occurs but is not captured by the myocardium

e. pacemaker does not recognize the patient's inherent heart rate

f. electrical current from muscle movements or other activities are sensed by the pacemaker

g. pacemaker fails to send electrical impulse to the heart

h. patient's own heart and the electronic pacemaker compete over electrical control of the heart

What Would You Do?

Read the following situations and use your critical thinking skills to determine how you would handle each. Write your answer in detail in the space provided.

39. When performing an ECG on Mr. Bobela, you notice chaotic electrical activity on the ECG tracing. Mr. Bobela was awake when you started the ECG and is lying quietly now. What should you do?

_____

_____

40. Ms. Gomez has a second degree AV block, Mobitz I rhythm. Mrs. Jenwren has a second degree AV block, Mobitz II. Which patient has a more serious condition? Explain your answer.

_____

_____

41. The rhythm on the ECG machine is ventricular tachycardia. What information would you need to know about the patient in order for proper treatment to begin?

_____

_____

42. You noticed that Mr. Green is having a wide QRS complex on the monitor. The continuous monitoring equipment has only three lead wires. How would you describe the type of block the patient is experiencing when notifying the physician of the change?

_____

_____

43. Mrs. Estes, an in-patient in your facility, has just finished shopping on the TV shopping network and knows that she has spent too much money. She is complaining that she is having palpitations. You notice that the heart rate is fast and her rhythm indicates an SVT pattern. What should you find out about the patient prior to notifying the licensed practitioner of the rapid heartbeat?

_____

_____

GET CONNECTED TO THE WEB

Cardiac Arrhythmias For information regarding cardiac arrhythmias (dysrhythmias) refer to Cardiac Electrophysiology Department of Inland Cardiology Associates, Spokane, WA, at http://www.iea.com/~epace/index.html. Once you have entered this site, click on the word *arrhythmias* and write down the list of symptoms of arrhythmia provided. If a patient has these symptoms, do they definitely have an arrhythmia?

Reviewing ECGs The 12-Lead ECG Library, at http://homepages.enterprise.net/djenkins/ecghome.html, is a great site for reviewing ECGs. Go to this site and study the rhythms before completing the rhythm identification review section in this chapter. In addition, find a dysrhythmia identified in this chapter review and write a description of it including the criteria for classification.

Rhythm Identification: Review the dysrhythmias pictured here and, using the criteria for classification provided in the chapter as clues, identify each rhythm and explain what information you used to make your decision.

46.

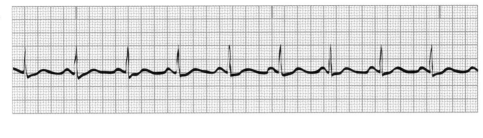

_____

_____

_____

_____

47.

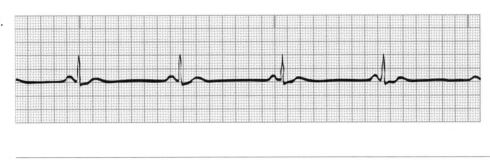

_____

_____

_____

_____

48.

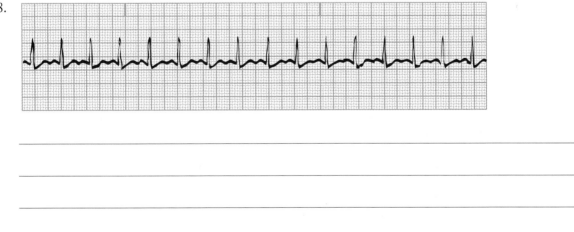

_____

_____

_____

_____

49.

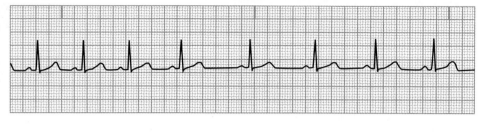

_____

_____

_____

50.

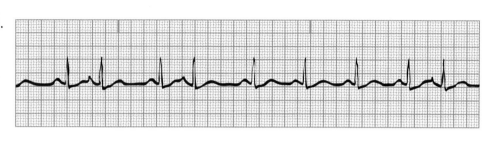

_____

_____

_____

51.

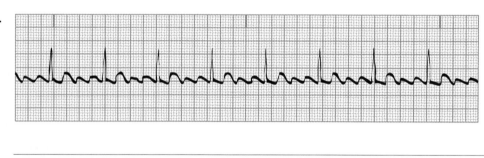

_____

_____

_____

52.

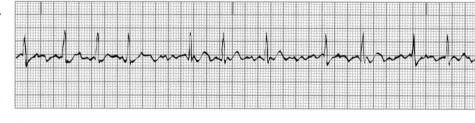

_____

_____

_____

53.

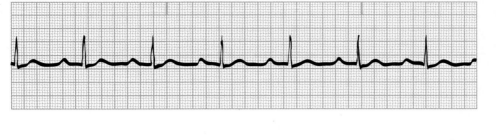

_____

_____

_____

54.

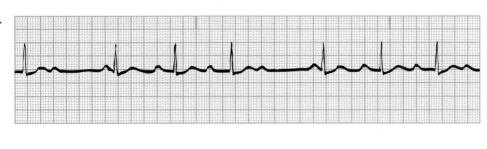

_____

_____

_____

55.

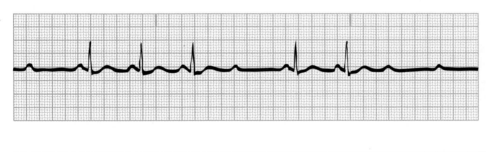

_____

_____

_____

56.

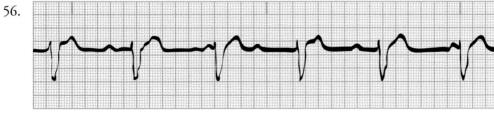

_____

_____

_____

57.

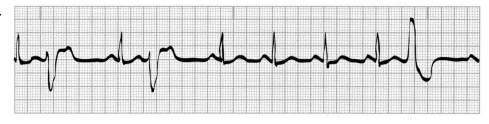

58.

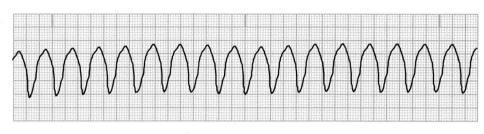

59.

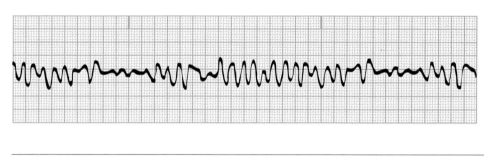

60.

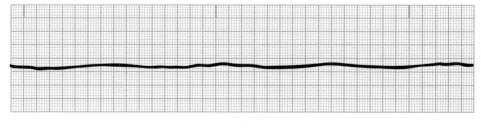

61.

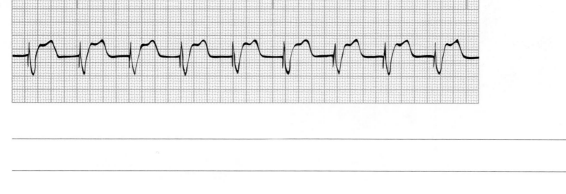

_____

_____

_____

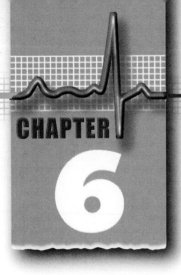

CHAPTER 6

Exercise Electrocardiography

Chapter Outline

- What Is Exercise Electrocardiography? (pg. 113)
- Why Is Exercise Electrocardiography Used? (pg. 114)
- Variations of Exercise Electrocardiography (pg. 114)
- Preparing and Educating the Patient (pg. 115)
- Providing Safety (pg. 118)
- Performing Exercise Electrocardiography (pg. 119)
- Following Exercise Electrocardiography (pg. 120)

Objectives

Upon completion of this chapter, you should be able to:

- ▌ Describe exercise electrocardiography.
- ▌ Identify at least three other names for exercise electrocardiography.
- ▌ List the different uses of exercise electrocardiography.
- ▌ Describe at least one variation of exercise electrocardiography.
- ▌ Prepare a patient for exercise electrocardiography.
- ▌ Perform patient teaching for exercise electrocardiography.
- ▌ List responsibilities of a health care giver for exercise electrocardiography.
- ▌ Understand and perform proper safety measures before, during, and after exercise electrocardiography.

Key Terms

angina - Pain around the heart radiating to the arm, caused by lack of oxygen to the heart muscle.

angiogram - An invasive procedure during which X-rays are taken of a blood vessel after injection of a radiopaque substance.

beta blockers - Drugs used to treat hypertension.

cardiologist - A physician who specializes in the study of the heart.

congestive heart failure - Failure of the heart to pump an adequate amount of blood to the body tissue.

coronary artery disease - Accumulation of plaque and fatty deposits in the coronary arteries that supply blood to the heart.

echocardiogram - Noninvasive diagnostic test that uses sound to study the heart and blood vessels; also known as an ultrasound.

false positive - When a diagnostic test indicates the presence of disease but in reality the test is negative and no disease is present.

hypertension - High blood pressure.

hyperventilate - To breathe at an increased rate and depth of inspiration and expiration.

invasive - Procedure that requires entrance into a body cavity, tissue, or blood vessel.

noninvasive - Procedure that does not require entrance into a body cavity, tissue, or blood vessel.

skin rasp - A rough piece of material used to abrade (scrape) the skin prior to electrode placement.

target heart rate (THR) - Heart rate measurement needed to truly exercise the heart; determined by subtracting the patient's age from 220.

thallium stress test - An invasive type of exercise electrocardiography in which thallium, a radiopaque substance (one that is visible with an X-ray machine) is injected into the body to permit viewing the vessels around the heart.

What Is Exercise Electrocardiography?

Often a patient has symptoms of cardiac problems that do not show up on a resting ECG. In order to determine the problems and to perform an accurate diagnosis, the physician may order an exercise electrocardiograph. Exercise electrocardiography has been used for more than fifty years. This test is known by many names, such as an exercise tolerance test, a treadmill stress test, a cardiac stress test, a stress ECG, or an exercise treadmill test. It is most commonly known as a treadmill stress test because the exercise is usually performed on an exercise treadmill (see Figure 6-1). This **noninvasive** procedure—meaning that it does not require entrance into a body cavity, tissue, or blood vessel—is an effective means of diagnosing cardiac disorders. The procedure is performed with a cardiologist or other physician present. The patient is carefully monitored throughout the testing.

During the procedure the patient is asked to walk on a treadmill, pedal an exercise bike, or climb a set of stairs (see Figure 6-2). While the person is exercising, an ECG is performed. The person is asked to increase the level of exertion of exercise as the test progresses. In addition to monitoring the ECG, the blood pressure, heart rate, skin temperature, oxygen level, and physical appearance are also assessed. The patient is asked to report any chest pain, dizziness, shortness of breath, or any other symptoms. Abnormalities, physical changes, or complaints could indicate a problem that requires treatment.

As a multiskilled health care provider, you will be responsible for providing patient instructions and monitoring the patient during the procedure by taking the blood pressure, observing for pain, discomfort, fatigue, or difficulty breathing, and applying and removing the electrodes. Your most important responsibility is to provide for safety and to be prepared in case an emergency should arise. The following is a list of your responsibilities during an exercise electrocardiograph.

- Provide for safety.
- Educate and prepare the patient prior to the procedure.
- Attach the electrodes properly.
- Instruct the patient to report symptoms.
- Monitor the patient, including blood pressure.

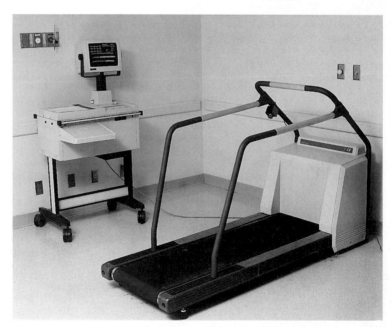

Figure 6-1: Common exercise electrocardiography equipment includes a treadmill, an ECG machine, and a monitor.

PATIENT EDUCATION AND COMMUNICATION - Failure to report an abnormal blood pressure or other complications such as tachycardia or increased respiration rate during exercise electrocardiography could lead to severe patient problems and inaccurate test results.

Why Is Exercise Electrocardiography Used?

Exercise electrocardiography is used to evaluate how the heart and blood vessels respond to physical activity. Treadmill stress testing is typically performed when the physician suspects a cardiac problem, most commonly coronary artery disease. **Coronary artery disease** is usually due to atherosclerosis, which occurs when plaque accumulates in the blood vessels. When the heart is exercised, it requires additional blood to provide oxygen to the myocardium (heart muscle). The exercise places an additional workload on the heart. If a patient has narrowed or obstructed arteries due to coronary artery disease, blood flow to the heart will not increase in response to the exercise. This additional workload may change the ECG tracing. One such change in the ECG tracing is ST segment depression, as shown in Figure 6-3. ST depression may indicate a myocardial infarction (MI). The exercise may also produce symptoms of chest pain (**angina**), weakness, shortness of breath, palpitations, or dizziness.

Exercise electrocardiography is used for other reasons as well. The physician may want to assess how well the

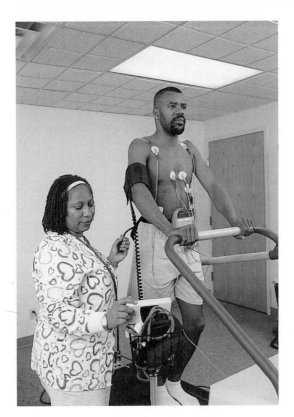

Figure 6-2: The goal during the treadmill test is to exercise the heart and evaluate how it responds to the stress of exercise.

patient's blood pressure is maintained during exercise. Exercise electrocardiography may also be used to evaluate exercise-induced symptoms such as palpitations or angina. It may also be performed to determine the patient's risk of a myocardial infarction. After an MI or cardiac surgery, the treadmill stress test is frequently used to evaluate the functioning of the heart. It may also be used to evaluate the effectiveness of cardiac medications, identify arrhythmias that occur during exercise, and aid in the development of an exercise program. The following is a list of uses for exercise electrocardiography.

- Helps diagnose cause of chest pain
- Determines functional capacity of the heart after surgery or myocardial infarction
- Screens for heart disease (particularly in men over age 35) when no symptoms are present
- Helps set limitations for an exercise program
- Identifies cause of abnormal heart rhythms that develop during physical exercise
- Evaluates effectiveness of heart medications

Variations of Exercise Electrocardiography

Figure 6-3: ST segment depression is depression of the ST segment below the normal baseline of the ECG. It indicates myocardial ischemia, which can occur during exercise electrocardiography.

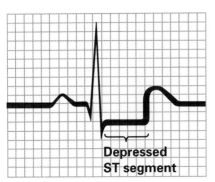

Depressed ST segment

One variation of exercise electrocardiography is a **thallium stress test.** A thallium stress test is similar to a treadmill stress test. The exercise and monitoring portion are the same; however, during a thallium stress test, the patient is injected intravenously with thallium one to two minutes before the end of the exercise period. Thallium is a radiopaque substance, which means it is visible to an X-ray machine. Thallium flows into the heart and is viewed by the **cardiologist,** a physician who specializes in the study of the heart, using a special camera or scanner. Taking pictures of the heart lasts about 10 to 20 minutes. The patient lies on a table with both arms above the head and the scanner above them. The heart is viewed immediately after the test as well as 3 to 4 hours later, when the patient has rested. The cardiologist studies the pictures to determine if blood flow to the heart improves with rest. Thallium flows more easily through nondiseased arteries. The purpose of the procedure is to determine if exercise causes a decrease in blood flow to any area of the heart. This procedure is considered **invasive** since the patient is injected with thallium.

Another variation of the exercise electrocardiography is a Persantine-thallium stress test. This test is similar to a thallium stress test with one exception: it is performed on patients who are not able to exercise. During this test, the physician or nurse administers medication called Persantine® (dipyridamole), which causes the heart to exercise artificially. The medication is injected over time to stimulate the heart to exercise throughout the testing. When Persantine and thallium are used in combination, this is known as a Persantine-thallium stress test. This test requires the patient to have intravenous injections of both thallium and Persantine.

Preparing and Educating the Patient

When scheduling a patient for exercise electocardiography, you will need to make sure the patient comes prepared for the test (see the checklist in Table 6-1). Describe the procedure and ensure that the patient understands. The patient should not smoke

Table 6-1 Exercise electrocardiography checklist

You can use a checklist such as this to provide documentation of patient instructions for the ambulatory monitoring procedure.

Exercise Electrocardiography—Checklist for Patient Education

Patient Name

Prior to the procedure the patient was able to:	YES	NO
■ Describe exercise electrocardiography		
■ Explain why the test is being performed		
■ Describe how exercise electrocardiography will be performed		
■ Wear comfortable clothing and shoes		
■ Avoid caffeine and tobacco 3 hours prior		
■ Eat a light meal at least 2 hours prior		
■ Name medications that should not be taken		
■ Explain the safety measures that will be used during the procedure		

During the procedure, the patient was able to:	YES	NO
■ Report symptoms or unusual occurrences		
■ Stop exercise when fatigued		

After the procedure, the patient understood:	YES	NO
■ Results are provided within 10 days by the physician		
■ He or she must rest for several hours		
■ Extreme temperature changes should be avoided		
■ Stimulants, such as caffeine, tobacco, or alcohol, should be avoided for at least 3 hours		
■ A hot shower or bath should be avoided for at least 3 hours		

Signature	Date	Initials

Table 6-2 Handling a patient's refusal to grant consent

Reason for Refusal	Possible Solution
Patient does not understand why the consent form is necessary	Explain the legal requirement of an informed consent and refer the patient to the physician for questions, if necessary
Patient does not understand the procedure	Notify the physician and provide a brochure for the patient to review while he or she is waiting for the physician to explain the procedure
Patient is illiterate and unable to sign his or her name	Have a witness present (preferably a family member) and have the consent form marked with an X by the patient and signed by the witness and yourself
Patient is unable to sign because glasses are not available	Make every attempt to obtain the glasses and then have the patient sign; if this is not possible, have the patient sign to the best of his or her ability; be certain to have a witness (preferably a family member) sign the form as well

or drink alcohol or caffeine three hours prior to the test. He or she should also be advised not to eat for at least two hours before the test. The patient should be instructed to bring or wear comfortable clothing and shoes. Tennis shoes and loose pants will make the exercise portion of the test easier for the patient.

Sometimes certain medications should not be taken prior to the test. You will need to instruct the patient regarding medications that should or should not be taken. Always check the physician's order. If it is not written on the chart or order, ask the physician. When asking, have a list of the patient's current medications or the patient's chart available for the physician to review. Medications commonly known as **beta blockers**—drugs used to treat hypertension—are frequently stopped prior to an exercise electrocardiograph because this type of medication could affect the test results or delay the test. Remember, your responsibility is to ensure that the patient comes to the office or clinic properly prepared for the exercise electrocardiograph.

A complete history of the patient may need to be recorded before beginning the test. A standard form should be used. The information you need to obtain from the patient includes the medical history, medications currently being taken, cardiovascular risk factors (see Table 1-1 in Chapter 1 on page 2), and the reason for this examination. Much of this information may already be on the patient's chart. In addition, a permission slip or informed consent form must be signed and witnessed (see Figure 6-4). The patient should understand the procedure, its risks, and the reason the test has been ordered before signing the informed consent form.

The patient should be informed that exercise electrocardiography is not a "timed" test. The length of time the test takes depends on several factors, including the

THE HEART INSTITUTE

PATIENT NAME (Print Clearly):_____

1. CONSENT TO TREATMENT: I (the above listed) consent to medical treatment by the physicians and staff of The Heart Institute.

2. FINANCIAL RESPONSIBILITY: I am aware that my account remains my responsibility. If insurance is filed, I will pay any unpaid balance after benefits have been determined or if no payment has been received after a reasonable period of time. I understand that payment in full is due within thirty (30) days after the first billing.

3. MEDICARE AUTHORIZATION: I request that payment of authorized Medicare payments be made either to me or on my behalf to The Heart Institute for any services furnished by that provider.

4. WORKER'S COMPENSATION CLAIMS: I am aware that I bear ultimate financial responsibility for all medical services rendered me by The Heart Institute. In the event that coverage is denied under Worker's compensation. I will pay any unpaid balance notwithstanding any appeal of denial.

5. MEDICAL RECORDS RELEASE: I, the undersigned, request any physician or hospital who have medical records concerning the above named patient to release a copy of the records to The Heart Institute. I also authorize the release of medical information to other physicians involved in my care or to my insurance company.

6. ATTORNEY SERVICES: I understand that in the event my bill is referred to an attorney for collection, I am responsible for all collection expenses, namely the attorney's fees in the amount of 33 1/3% of the total amount then due and court costs.

7. ABDOMINAL ULTRASOUND WAIVER: Medicare will only pay for services that it determines to be "reasonable and necessary" under section 1862 (A)(1) of the Medicare law. If Medicare determines that abdominal ultrasound isn't "reasonable and necessary" under Medicare program standards, Medicare will deny payment for that service. If Medicare or other insurance denies payment for abdominal ultrasound, I agree to be personally responsible for payment.

8. HOLTER MONITOR & AMBULATORY BLOOD PRESSURE MONITOR WAIVER: I understand that Medicare will only reimburse the use to Holter monitors every six months and Medicare and some companies do not cover 24-Hour Blood Pressure monitoring. When it is necessary to apply a Holter monitor more often than every six months or apply a B.P. monitor, I agree to these tests at my expense.

9. TELEPHONE CALL WAIVER: I understand that Medicare and some insurance companies do not cover telephone calls. If a telephone call lasts more than four minutes, I agree to pay for these calls at my expense.

10. HIV/HEPATITIS TESTING: In accordance with Virginia law, any patient to whose body fluids a health care worker has been exposed, and any health care worker to whose body fluids a patient has been exposed, will be deemed to have consented to HIV and HEPATITIS B or C testing. I understand that if my doctor has determined that it is necessary to test my/my child's blood for that antibody to the Human Immunodeficiency Virus, I agree to have HIV blood testing. I understand that if my or my child's HIV and/or Hepatitis B or C test result is positive, state law requires that this result be reported to the State Health Department.

Date:_____Patient Signature_____

Date of Birth_____Social Security Number:_____

*RESPONSIBLE PARTY OTHER THAN PATIENT: I agree to accept full financial responsibility for the account of the above named patient.

Responsible Party Signature:_____

Relationship:_____

Figure 6-4: Your patient must sign an informed consent for exercise electrocardiography. Most facilities use a standardized form such as the one pictured here.

patient's age, degree of conditioning or health status, other medical problems, and medications. You should inform the patient that the test will take approximately 45 minutes to an hour. Carefully explain the safety precautions provided during the procedure to help alleviate any fears the patient may have.

Providing Safety

Exercise electrocardiography is done on patients who are already at risk. At-risk patients may have just recently had a myocardial infarction or may currently be experiencing some type of chest pain or other symptoms, or they may have a history of coronary artery disease. Exercise electrocardiography does place stress on the patient's heart. There is some risk of a heart attack or stroke during the procedure that should be considered. You should follow the safety measures and be prepared for emergencies (see Table 6-3).

Table 6-3 Preparing for emergencies during exercise electrocardiography

- Inform the patient how he or she can expect to feel during the test, including mild fatigue, increased heart rate, perspiration, and increased breath rate.

- Explain to the patient the need to report signs and symptoms such as chest or other pain, dizziness, weakness, or extreme fatigue.

- Make sure the patient knows to stop the exercise if any pain or extreme fatigue is felt.

- Make sure the physician is present during the entire procedure.

- Check to see that emergency equipment is close by.

- Observe and monitor the patient and report any symptoms to the physician.

In order to provide for safety, certain rules must be followed. A physician should always be present during the procedure. Emergency equipment should be in the room or nearby, including a crash cart with emergency medications and supplies. You must know the location of this equipment. In addition, the patient should be monitored at all times and he or she must understand the need to report any abnormal symptoms when they occur.

Some health conditions prevent patients from participating in exercise electrocardiography. These conditions include, but are not limited to:

- heart aneurysm

- uncontrolled disturbances in the heartbeat

- inflammation surrounding the heart or heart muscle

- severe anemia

- uncontrolled **hypertension** (high blood pressure)

- unstable angina

- **congestive heart failure** (the heart's failure to pump an adequate volume of blood)

The physician should be aware of any of these conditions. Make sure that the health history is current and complete for the physician to review.

Performing Exercise Electrocardiography

Assemble and prepare the equipment before the patient's arrival. You will need:

- blood pressure equipment
- shaving equipment, abrasive skin cleaner, skin rasp
- alcohol solution
- cotton swabs
- chest electrodes
- electrode paste or gel (not necessary if electrodes are pregelled)
- ECG machine with monitor
- lead wires
- treadmill or stationary bicycle
- adhesive tape or rubber belt (used to attach monitoring unit)

When the patient arrives for the test, you should verify that he or she has come properly prepared by making sure the patient has not had alcohol, caffeine, or tobacco for at least three hours prior to the test. Verify that medications were stopped, if required. Complete the patient's medical history and make sure the informed consent form has been signed.

Next, prepare the electrode sites for placement. If the sites are hairy, dry shave the skin. Rub the site with an alcohol swab and let it dry. Abrade the skin using a special prep pad, dry 4 x 4 gauze, **skin rasp,** or other type of abrasive cleaner. Abrading the skin consists of rubbing firmly and briskly at each of the sites where the electrodes will be placed to ensure that they will adhere better to the skin.

Attach the blood pressure cuff and electrodes. Check the manufacturer's instructions for the system you are using and the policy at your facility for correct placement of the electrodes (see Figure 6-5). Some machines include a diagram that provides

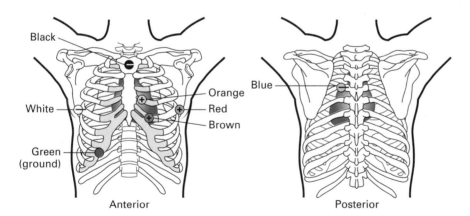

Figure 6-5: Standard placement of electrodes for exercise electrocardiography. Since machines may vary, check the manufacturer's instructions for proper placement of the electrodes for the exercise electrocardiograph machine you are using. As shown, electrodes are often placed on both chest and back for a better view of the electrical activity of the heart.

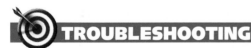

TROUBLESHOOTING

If your patient has any complaints or problems during exercise electrocardiography, you should be prepared to respond. Keep in mind that while the physician should be in the room, he or she may not always be aware of the patient's complaints or problems. Any symptom that the patient reports such as extreme fatigue, dizziness, shortness of breath, or chest pain should be immediately reported to the physician. If the patient collapses, you should check the pulse and respiration and begin emergency procedures as appropriate.

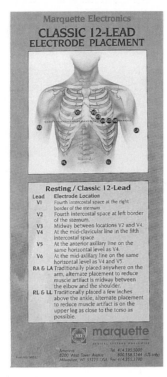

information for correct placement (see Figure 6-6). Most exercise electrocardiography monitors include leads for both chest and back.

Prior to the exercise, a resting ECG is performed and the blood pressure is taken to obtain a baseline. The patient is asked to breathe quickly and deeply (**hyperventilate**) for about 30 seconds and then another ECG and blood pressure reading are taken. The second ECG is done to identify ECG changes that occur as a result of changes in breathing. These changes could be misinterpreted as being related to heart disease if they occurred during the treadmill exam.

The test is divided into stages of two or three minutes each. The physician determines the specific length of each stage of exercise. The entire exercise period lasts up to 15 minutes. The time may vary based on the patient's cardiac risk factors and ability. At the end of each stage, the patient's blood pressure is checked, the ECG is repeated, and the level of exercise is increased.

Most people walk or ride to the point of fatigue or symptoms of chest discomfort or shortness of breath. The supervising physician may halt the test because of blood pressure, ECG, or heart rhythm changes that are not perceived by the patient. In other words, though the patient may not complain of any symptoms, the physician may identify changes in the blood pressure, heart rate, or ECG tracing that may lead to complications and may order that the test be stopped.

During the test, the goal is to achieve the **target heart rate** (THR) without symptoms or complications. The target heart rate is two hundred and twenty (220) minus the patient's age. This is different from the target heart rate for aerobic exercise, which is only 60% to 80% of this number. The THR is the rate that the patient should not be allowed to exceed during the test. Achieving the target heart rate without symptoms or abnormalities is a good indication that the heart is functioning well. Generally, the closer the patient is to the target heart rate, the more reliable the results are.

Instruct the patient to report any symptoms such as shortness of breath, chest pain, dizziness, or weakness they experience during the procedure because you are responsible for monitoring and recording this information (see Figure 6-7). You will need to monitor blood pressure, pulse, and any signs of cardiac distress. You may also be monitoring the patient's blood oxygen level on the monitor screen. Watch the patient closely including skin color, breathing pattern, amount of perspiration, and facial expressions. Many times a patient is hesitant to report a symptom. If you suspect a problem, ask the patient and then report your suspicion to the supervising physician.

> **PATIENT EDUCATION AND COMMUNICATION** - You can help reduce the patient's fears by maintaining a sense of confidence, answering questions, and following safety precautions during exercise electrocardiography.

Following Exercise Electrocardiography

When the patient has completed the exercise portion of the test, monitoring will continue during a "cooling off" period. This will last approximately 10 to 15 minutes. You will need to stay with the patient and continue to monitor the patient for any changes.

THE HEART INSTITUTE

EXERCISE TEST

Predicted maximal heart rate for age:_____

Exercise Performed	Min.	HR	BP	COMMENTS	INTERPRETATION
Resting-Strip #1					
Stage I - Strip #2 2 mph 10% Grade	1				
	2				
Stage II - Strip #3 3 mph 10% Grade	3				
	4				
Stage III - Strip #4 4 mph 10% Grade	5				
	6				
Stage IV - Strip #5 5 mph 10% Grade	7				
	8				
Recovery Strip # 6 5 min.					
Patient:			Age:		Date:

Medications: Conclusion:

Fluoroscopy:

Oliver D. White, Jr. M.D.

Many factors are used to interpret the results of exercise electrocardiography. The most important factors are the presence of ECG changes and symptoms. Other factors include heart rate and rhythm, blood pressure, and changes in oxygen consumption. If a patient has no abnormal ECG changes or unusual elevations in blood pressure, this usually means the risk for coronary artery disease is low. If the test is stopped early because of ECG or blood pressure changes or patient symptoms, this is a sign of abnormal test results. When the results of the test are inconclusive or abnormal, additional tests may be performed. An inconclusive test is one with questionable results, meaning it does not necessarily show an abnormality or eliminate the potential for an abnormality. Additional testing is needed to either identify or eliminate any abnormalities. These additional tests may include an **echocardiogram,** which uses sound to study the heart and blood vessels (also known as ultrasound), or a coronary **angiogram,** involving X-rays following injection of a radiopaque substance.

PATIENT EDUCATION AND COMMUNICATION - As a multiskilled health care giver, you are not responsible for reporting the results of exercise electrocardiography to the patient. Should a question arise, refer the patient to the physician.

After exercise electrocardiography the patient should be given some instructions. These include:

- Rest for several hours.
- Avoid extreme temperature changes.
- Avoid stimulants, such as caffeine, tobacco, or alcohol, for at least 3 hours.
- Do not take a hot shower or bath for at least 2 hours.
- Do not expect results of the examination for up to 10 days: discuss the results with your physician when available.

Stress testing is considered a good method to detect early coronary artery disease and delay its progression. However, it is interesting to note that approximately 5% of healthy adults may have **false positive** results, meaning that the test may indicate that disease is present when it is not. Research has shown that false positives occur more frequently in females than in males, though researchers are not sure why. False positives can cause unnecessary fears and the need for additional expensive tests.

Chapter Review

It's Your Choice: Circle the correct answer for each of the following.

1. What is your most important responsibility during exercise electrocardiography?

   a. providing for safety

   b. applying the leads

   c. monitoring the ECG tracing

   d. taking the patient's blood pressure

2. Which of the following conditions would be a reason that a patient should not perform exercise electrocardiography?

   a. coronary artery disease

   b. previous heart attack

   c. congestive heart failure

   d. previous symptoms of angina

3. What type of test would be performed on a patient who is unable to stand or exercise?

   a. thallium stress test

   b. Persantine-thallium test

   c. treadmill stress test

   d. cardiac stress test

4. During exercise electrocardiography, your patient appears to be short of breath. After informing the physician of your suspicions, what would you do?

   a. continue the test

   b. take the patient's blood pressure

   c. ask the patient to stop the exercise portion of the test

   d. without the patient's knowledge, count the respiratory rate and compare to the previous rate

5. Mr. Jones is on several medications and is scheduled for an exercise electrocardiograph tomorrow. What should you do first to determine if he should take his medications prior to the test?

   a. check the chart or order

   b. ask the physician

   c. instruct the patient not to take his beta blocker medications

   d. Mr. Jones should take all of his medications since they are necessary for his treatment

Test Your Patient Education Techniques: You are assigned to teach Mr. Hussein about exercise electrocardiography. From the list below, determine which are correct patient instructions for exercise electrocardiography and which are not. Place a *C* beside the correct statements and an *I* beside the incorrect statements. For each of the incorrect (I) statements, write the correct instructions for the patient.

_____ 6. Patients should avoid alcohol, tobacco, and caffeine for at least 8 hours prior to exercise electrocardiography.

_____

_____

_____ 7. Patients should be encouraged to report any symptoms such as shortness of breath, weakness, dizziness, or fatigue during exercise electrocardiography.

_____

_____

_____ **8.** After exercise electrocardiography the patient should not take a hot bath or shower for at least 2 hours.

_____

_____

_____ **9.** You should discuss the results of exercise electrocardiography with the patient as soon as they are available.

_____

_____

_____ **10.** Patients should wear comfortable, casual clothing on the day of the test including tennis shoes and loose fitting pants.

_____

_____

_____ **11.** You should attach the leads to the chest at the same sites as you would for an ambulatory monitor.

_____

_____

_____ **12.** Emergency equipment should be available in the room or nearby during exercise electrocardiography.

_____

_____

Leading Edge Lead Placement: Label the correct electrode placement for exercise electrocardiography.

Anterior   Posterior

13. _____

14. _____

15. _____

16. _____

17. _____

18. _____

19. _____

The Match Game: Match these terms with the correct definitions. Place the appropriate letter on the line to the left of each term.

_____ 20. thallium stress test

_____ 21. myocardium

_____ 22. hypertension

_____ 23. beta blocker

_____ 24. angiogram

_____ 25. angina

_____ 26. arrhythmia

_____ 27. cardiologist

_____ 28. congestive heart failure

_____ 29. coronary artery disease

_____ 30. echocardiogram

_____ 31. false positive

_____ 32. THR

_____ 33. invasive

_____ 34. noninvasive

a. medication used to treat hypertension
b. pain around the heart caused by lack of oxygen to the heart
c. failure of the heart to pump an adequate amount of blood to the tissue
d. loss of normal rhythm of the heart beat
e. a physician who specializes in the study of the heart
f. X-rays taken of the blood vessels after injection of a radiopaque substance
g. accumulation of plaque and fatty deposits in the coronary arteries
h. noninvasive diagnostic test that uses ultrasound to study the heart and blood vessels
i. when a diagnostic test indicates that disease is present and in reality the test is negative
j. high blood pressure
k. requires entrance into a body cavity, tissue, or blood vessel to be completed
l. middle layer of the heart composed of muscle tissue
m. procedure that does _not_ require entrance into a body cavity, tissue, or blood vessel
n. calculated by subtracting your age from 220
o. exercise electrocardiography that is invasive because of injection of a radiopaque substance to view the vessels around the heart

What Would You Do?

Read the following situations and use your critical thinking skills to determine how you would handle each. Write your answer in detail in the space provided.

35. Your patient, Mr. Rollins, is scheduled for an exercise electrocardiograph on Friday. When scheduling the appointment, you notice he is taking several heart medications including Atenolol. You check the patient's order and it does not mention whether any of the medications should not be taken before the procedure. Mr. Rollins is getting ready to leave. What should you do?

_____

_____

36. During an exercise electrocardiography procedure your patient complains of weakness and shortness of breath. He suddenly collapses on the treadmill and falls into the chair. What should you do?

_____

_____

37. Mrs. Annon just had an exercise electrocardiogram performed. You are responsible for providing instructions to her before she leaves. After you review the instructions, Mrs. Annon tells you she is going to go for a walk to have a cigarette while she waits for her husband to pick her up. It is about 97 degrees outside. What should you do?

_____

_____

38. Mr. Wong is required to have a thallium stress test at the outpatient clinic where you are employed. He is a very busy businessman and requests to have the test during his lunch hour. What would be your response?

_____

_____

GET CONNECTED TO THE WEB

Patient Information for Exercise Electrocardiography The following three sites all provide patient information regarding exercise electrocardiography. Review these sites and search for other websites to research how frequently exercise electrocardiography is performed and its effectiveness. Be prepared to present your information to the class or prepare your own patient informational brochure.
- Mayo Health Exercise Stress Test:
  http://www.mayohealth.org/mayo/9411/htm/stresste.htm
- Thrive on Line Health Library:
  http://www.thriveonline.com/health/Library/medtests/medtest174.html
- The Virtual Hospital Treadmill Electrocardiogram:
  http://vh.radiology.uiowa.edu/Patients/IHB/IntMed/Cardio/TreadmillEKG.html

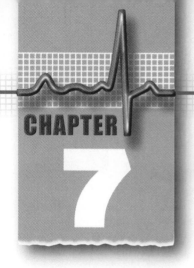

CHAPTER 7

Ambulatory Monitoring

Objectives

Upon completion of this chapter, you will be able to:

▶ Identify the different types of ambulatory monitors and their functions

▶ Identify variations of Holter monitoring

▶ Explain why ambulatory monitoring is used in addition to the 12-lead ECG

▶ List the common uses for ambulatory monitoring

▶ Educate the patient about ambulatory monitoring

▶ Prepare a patient for application of an ambulatory monitor

▶ Apply and remove an ambulatory monitor correctly

▶ Identify the procedure for reporting the results from ambulatory monitoring

Key Terms

ambulate - To walk.

anti-arrhythmic - Type of medication given to prevent arrhythmias.

arrhythmia - Irregularity or loss of rhythm of the heartbeat.

Holter - Proper name given to one type of ambulatory monitor, named after Norman Holter, inventor of the procedure and machine.

oscilloscope - A monitor or TV-type device used to view the tracing of the heart or ECG.

palpitation - Fast heartbeat sensation felt by the patient, which may or may not be associated with complaints of chest pain.

stress ECG - Another name for exercise electrocardiography.

syncope - Fainting spells.

What Is Ambulatory Monitoring?

Ambulatory monitoring is the process of recording an ECG tracing for an extended period of time while a patient goes about his or her daily activities, including walking or **ambulating.** A typical ambulatory monitor is a small box that is strapped to the patient's waist or shoulder to record an ECG over a 24- to 48-hour period (see Figure 7-1). Inside the box is a recording device; the entire device usually weighs less than two pounds. The most common type looks like a small tape recorder. Newer ambulatory monitors on the market are digital

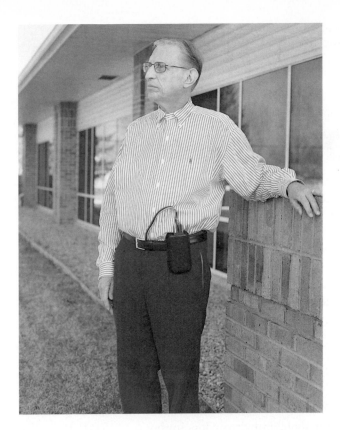

Figure 7-1: An ambulatory monitor is attached to the shoulder or waist so the patient is free to move about during the 24- to 48-hour period while the electrical activity of the heart is being recorded.

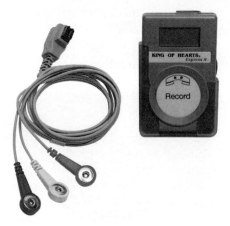

Figure 7-2: The newer digital ambulatory monitors record the electrical activity of the heart, which can be transferred directly to a computer for interpretation.

recorders, as seen in Figure 7-2. One type of ambulatory monitor is also known as a **Holter** monitor, named after its inventor, Norman Holter.

During ambulatory monitoring, the patient has 3 to 5 leads attached to his or her chest, depending on the type of monitor used. The patient may move around and is encouraged to maintain his or her normal daily activities. While the monitor is in place and recording, the patient is asked to keep a diary to record all usual and unusual activities. Any symptoms or abnormal sensations such as chest pain, indigestion, or dizziness should be recorded. If symptoms do occur, the patient is asked to note the symptoms and what he or she was doing prior to and during the symptoms. When the monitoring is completed, the information from the monitor and diary must be interpreted. A computer is used to print and/or view the ECG tracing from the monitor. A computer may be used for analysis of the tracing. This computer analysis may be done within the facility, or the tracing may be sent to an outside laboratory, known as a reference laboratory. A physician, usually a cardiologist, does final interpretation of the results. If the results are sent to a reference laboratory, they are returned to the patient's physician.

As a multiskilled health care provider, you will be responsible for applying and removing the ambulatory monitor, providing patient education, and ensuring that the results are placed in the patient's chart. Depending on your place of employment, you may be responsible for attaching the tape to a machine called a scanner. The scanner will analyze the results and provide a printout for the physician to interpret.

How Is Ambulatory Monitoring Used?

The purpose of ambulatory monitoring is to document the electrical activity in the heart and identify any abnormal heart behaviors such as dysrhythmias. Abnormal heart behaviors can occur randomly or spontaneously and may be sleep related, disease related, or stress induced. As you have learned in previous chapters, abnormal electrical behavior of the heart can be life threatening.

An ambulatory monitor is used to capture abnormal heart rhythms and correlate symptoms experienced by the patient. For example, a typical patient may be experiencing chest pain, lightheadedness, **syncope** (fainting spells), dizziness, or

palpitations (rapid heartbeat). To find the cause of these symptoms, the patient may have already had a 12-lead ECG and a cardiac **stress ECG** (exercise electrocardiogram). However, the patient may not have experienced symptoms during these tests, so no abnormal rhythms would have been detected. If the patient is still having symptoms, an ambulatory monitor can be used. During the 24 to 48 hours that the monitor is in place, the patient records all daily activities, abnormal experiences, and symptoms in a diary. The ambulatory monitor provides an ECG tracing at the exact time the patient experiences any symptoms. The physician can interpret the results and evaluate the patient's symptoms based on the ECG tracing.

Ambulatory monitoring is used for other reasons as well. The physician may want to evaluate the effectiveness of cardiac medications such as **anti-arrhythmic** drug therapy (medication given to prevent arrhythmias). Ambulatory monitoring is also used to evaluate artificial pacemaker functioning. Pacemaker functioning is evaluated after implantation or if problems arise. Ambulatory monitoring can also evaluate the function of the heart after a recent myocardial infarction.

Functions and Variations

The two most common types of ambulatory monitoring are continuous and intermittent. Continuous monitoring provides a complete tracing of the ECG from the time the monitor is applied until it is removed. During continuous monitoring, the patient may be asked to press a button on the machine to mark the tracing whenever a symptom is felt. This is known as an "event marker." The marker marks the tracing at the exact time the event occurs. The monitor has an accurate clock that indicates the time the marker is applied. The clock is necessary for the physician to be able to correlate the diary entries with what is happening on the ECG tracing.

Intermittent recording records only while the patient is experiencing symptoms. The patient is instructed to press a button on the machine when symptoms occur to start the ECG tracing. The results from this type of tracing are shorter and can be evaluated more quickly than continuous monitoring. However, intermittent monitoring only shows the ECG tracing during the symptoms. Some abnormal rhythms can occur prior to symptoms, and an intermittent recording may not show these abnormalities.

Some ambulatory monitors can be voice activated. When the patient experiences an unusual symptom or changes in activity, he or she can speak into the recorder to describe each event. The event is timed for comparison to the ECG tracing during continuous monitoring. During intermittent monitoring, the ECG tracing may also be activated by the voice. (It is your responsibility to know the type and features of the monitor used in order to properly apply, remove, and instruct the patient.)

Some physicians prefer to use a 12-lead Holter monitoring system. As you already know, most ambulatory monitoring systems record only one lead tracing using a 3- or 5-lead system. In Chapter 3 you learned that a 12-lead ECG usually requires 10 lead wires and electrodes. Newer Holter monitoring systems have been developed using 5 leads to record a 12-lead tracing during the Holter monitoring. These systems provide more accurate and complete results because they record the 12 different views of the heart during the monitoring period.

Two other variations of ambulatory monitoring include telemetry and transtelephonic monitoring. Telemetry monitoring is performed within a medical facility such as a hospital, whereas transtelephonic monitoring is performed outside the medical facility. Both of these types of monitoring are performed on patients who can ambulate.

SAFETY AND INFECTION CONTROL - Ambulatory monitors are sensitive and can be very expensive. Be careful when handling an ambulatory monitor. Dropping or hitting the machine against something could cause permanent damage.

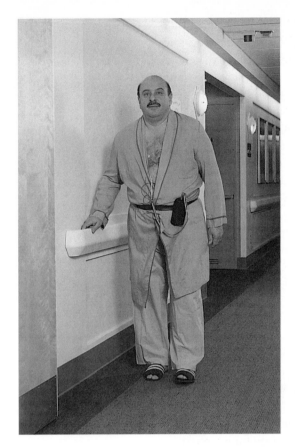

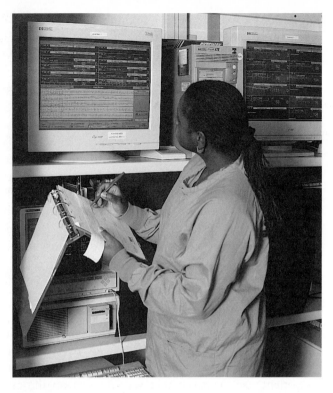

Figure 7-4: On a telemetry cardiac care unit, several patients can be monitored simultaneously at a central patient care station.

Figure 7-3: On the telemetry unit of an inpatient facility, patients wear the telemetry monitor leads and the unit attached to the chest and strapped around the shoulder or waist. This allows patients to ambulate and perform activities of daily living during their hospitalization.

Telemetry monitoring is done with a small transmitting device attached to the chest with three or five electrodes (see Figure 7-3). A continuous tracing of the heart is recorded and sent directly to a monitoring station. Telemetry monitors are only transmitting devices designed to send the electrical signal of the heart to a central location to be evaluated continuously. At this location, single or multiple patients may be monitored at the same time on multiple screens (see Figure 7-4). There is no need for a patient diary since the patient is admitted to the facility and will be observed and monitored at all times. In a cardiac intensive care unit, your role as a multiskilled health care giver may include observing the ECG tracings for abnormalities on a computer-type screen known as an **oscilloscope** (see Figure 7-5). You will need to be familiar with the **arrhythmias** (irregularities in heartbeat) presented in Chapter 5. In addition, you may also be required to pass a certification examination to work as a telemetry monitoring technician.

Transtelephonic monitoring was developed in the 1960s, after Holter monitoring was developed. It is used mainly to evaluate pacemaker function but is also used for any patient requiring monitoring for longer

Figure 7-5: The cardiac intensive care single oscilloscope allows you to view the ECG tracings for patients in a cardiac care unit.

than 24 to 48 hours. Patients with permanent pacemakers or certain cardiac dysrhythmias may require monitoring for 30 days or more. Transtelephonic monitors are small and portable. The information recorded is stored in the monitor and later transmitted over the telephone line (see Figure 7-6).

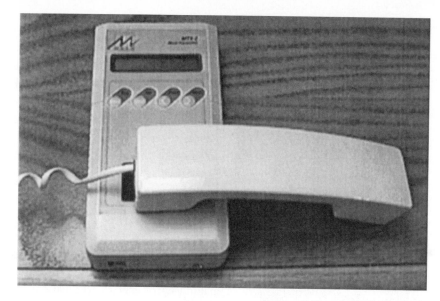

Figure 7-6: Transtelephonic monitors are attached to the telephone, then the information is transmitted to a health care facility for interpretation.

There are two types of transtelephonic monitors. One type is known as a postsymptom event monitor. This type is used when a patient is experiencing symptoms. It is worn like a wristwatch or it can be handheld. The handheld type should be kept in a convenient place by the patient and is activated when pressed onto the chest. The patient should activate the monitor while experiencing symptoms. The electrode feet on the handheld monitor record a lead II tracing (Figure 7-7). The wristwatch type is worn at all times and records a two-directional or bipolar lead I tracing. Postsymptom event monitoring records the heart activity for short periods immediately after the patient experiences symptoms. It is used primarily to document arrhythmias that last more than a few seconds, such as atrial fibrillation, atrial flutter, and supraventricular tachycardias.

Another type of transtelephonic monitor is a loop-memory monitor. This small device is attached to the chest with two lead wires. It remains in place continuously throughout the monitoring period, which may be 30 days or more. The memory on this monitor can hold up to five minutes of the ECG tracing and is programmed based on the patient's symptoms and complaints. For example, if a patient has a history of syncope (fainting spells), activating the monitor after an episode will lock the previous five minutes of ECG tracing into the memory for transmission over the telephone and evaluation. This provides the physician with an ECG tracing of the heart before, during, and after the episode and helps the physician determine the cause of the syncope.

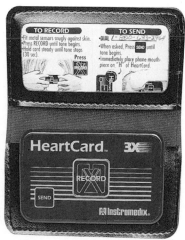

Figure 7-7. The small Heart Card monitor is activated by the patient when pressed onto the chest.

TROUBLESHOOTING

Sometimes during ambulatory monitoring the electrodes may become loose or disconnect and the patient will need to know how to handle this situation. Check the policy of the facility where you are employed to give the patient correct instructions. Usually patients are instructed to press loose electrodes in the center to reapply. However, if the electrode comes off completely, the patient will need to report this and return to the facility for replacement. Information about how and when to contact your place of employment should be provided to the patient.

Educating the Patient

PATIENT EDUCATION AND
COMMUNICATION - Begin by
asking the patient to tell you what
he or she already knows about the
ambulatory monitoring procedure.
Based on their response, you can
then explain to them what they do
not know or understand. This is an
effective way to ensure that your
patient understands the procedure.
You should also have the patient
repeat the information back to you
to demonstrate his or her
understanding.

Prior to having an ambulatory monitor, the patient must be thoroughly instructed on its proper use. Maintaining a diary is vital for accurate interpretation and evaluation of the results of the ECG tracing. The ECG tracing alone is not helpful unless the physician can correlate the results with the activities and symptoms the patient was experiencing during the tracing. Your responsibility is to ensure that the patient understands the monitoring procedure, why it is being done, and what he or she must do while the monitor is in place.

The Patient Diary

The patient diary must be an accurate record of the events and symptoms that occur while the monitor is in place (see Figure 7-8). Most diaries provide time blocks to mark when activities and symptoms occur, making entry easy for the patient (see Figure 7-9). The patient must record *all* activities, including physical and emotional stress and all usual and unusual daily events, such as urinating, bowel movements, sexual activities, walking, emotional upset, eating, and sleeping. You should emphasize the need for an accurate and complete diary. Make sure the patient knows not to change diet or daily activity during ambulatory monitoring.

To ensure that the patient understands the diary recording procedure, have him or her repeat your instructions back to you. You may want the patient to demonstrate his or her understanding by placing a sample entry into the diary. If the patient does not understand how to maintain the diary correctly, the monitoring procedure may have to be repeated. This unnecessary time and expense can be avoided by properly instructing the patient.

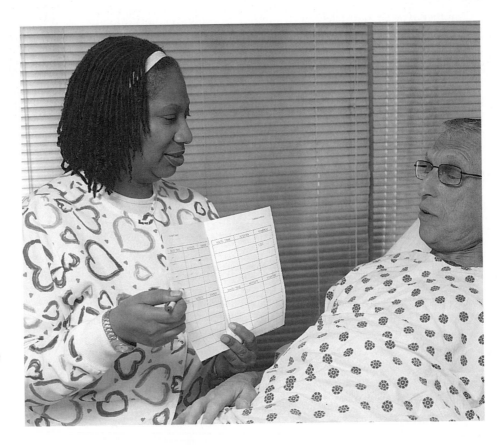

Figure 7-8: Explain the importance of the patient diary and the need for an accurate account of the patient's activities during the monitoring. Make sure the patient understands the diary's importance before he or she leaves with an ambulatory monitor.

Sample Diary

A portion of a sample diary is shown below. Remember that the more complete your diary, the more value it is for your doctor. If in doubt, write it down. Please print clearly so that your doctor or technician will understand your comments.

TIME	ACTIVITY	SYMPTOM
11:30 am	walking in hall	dizzy
1:45 pm	BM	
2:30 pm	exercise class began	
3:45 pm	sitting watching TV	flutter
11:30	Bed	

Patient Instructions

Carry this diary and a pencil with you at all times and enter your activities, symptoms, and times they occur. Generally you should record:

Time of Day: For every entry in the diary.

Activities: Routine & strenuous exercise, bowel movements, taking medication, or emotional upsets, such as anger.

Symptoms: Chest, neck, arm or face pain, heart pounding, dizziness, nausea, shortness of breath or any other–whether or not you feel they are important. If in doubt, write it down.

Important:
1. Do not tamper with the recorder, electrodes, or electrode leads.
2. Do not get the recorder wet.
3. Your recorder is equipped with a digital clock display and an event marker button; activate it when symptoms occur.

Patient Activity Diary

( )hr   ( )12 hr   ( )24 hr

Patient's Name_____
Patient's Addr._____

_____

Age:_____ Sex:_____
Phone:_____
Medication:_____

_____

Hospital:_____
Room:_____
Date of Recording:_____
Started:_____am/pm
Connected by:_____

_____

Figure 7-9: Note the sample entries in this Holter monitoring patient diary. The patient should make entries into this diary frequently throughout the Holter monitoring period.

As previously mentioned, ambulatory (Holter) monitoring may be done to evaluate the effectiveness of new cardiac medications or the patient's response to discontinuation of cardiac medications. In these circumstances, the physician may change the patient's heart medications prior to the monitoring, either adding a new medication or discontinuing one the patient is currently taking. It is your responsibility to remind the patient of medication changes prescribed by the physician.

It is best that the patient wear loose-fitting clothing during the monitoring procedure for comfort and convenience. A front-buttoning shirt is preferred because you can conveniently access the patient's chest and apply the electrodes. The patient must not tamper with the monitor or disconnect the lead wires or electrodes. While the monitor is in place, he or she may take only a sponge bath; no shower or tub bath is allowed during the monitoring because the equipment must not get wet. Patients may sleep in any position that does not apply tension on the lead wires or electrodes. Avoiding magnets, metal detectors, high-voltage areas and electric blankets is necessary because these devices can interfere with the tracing. The patient should also know how the monitoring equipment works and be instructed to check that it is working properly during the procedure. Documentation of

LAW AND ETHICS - Licensed practitioners are responsible for educating the patient regarding actions, indications, side effects, and precautions of medications. When a question arises regarding this information, refer the patient to a licensed practitioner to avoid practicing outside the scope of your education and training.

TROUBLESHOOTING

When reviewing the instructions for the diary with your patient, he asks you if he is allowed to do certain things during the monitoring such as sleep on his stomach or dance at an upcoming dinner party. You should inform him that he is encouraged to participate in his normal daily activities during the monitoring, whatever they may be. Since there is a chance that some activities may cause the electrodes to become loose or disconnected, you should check to be sure he knows the procedure for correcting this situation. You should also explain that if the electrodes become loose or disconnected, it could interfere with the accuracy of the results.

accurate patient education is necessary and must be included on the patient's chart (see Table 7-1).

Table 7-1 **Ambulatory monitoring checklist**		
You can use a checklist such as this to provide documentation of patient instructions for the ambulatory monitoring procedure.		
Ambulatory Monitoring—Checklist for Patient Education		
Patient Name		
Patient was able to:	**YES**	**NO**
■ Describe ambulatory monitoring		
■ Explain why he or she is having the test performed		
■ Know the length of time the monitor will be on		
■ State where the leads are placed and what they will feel like		
■ Adjust the shoulder strap or waist belt		
■ Wear appropriate clothing for comfort and convenience		
■ Take a sponge bath only		
■ Replace loose electrodes and report loose or removed electrodes		
■ Avoid metal detectors, electric detectors, high-voltage wires, and magnets		
■ Log usual and unusual activities and symptoms experienced		
Signature	**Date**	**Initials**

Preparing the Patient

Patients must be prepared for the ambulatory monitoring procedure both emotionally and physically. Many times the patient will be apprehensive. Children may be especially fearful. The first step in reducing the fear is to help them understand the procedure. Take time with the patient to explain each step of the procedure as you perform it. For children, be sure to explain in terms they can understand. Let the patient know it is normal to have some fear and allow the patient to express his or her feelings. Allow the patient to ask questions, and answer as completely as you can. If you do not know the answer, ask a licensed practitioner or your supervisor.

The patient should understand the physical requirements of the monitoring procedure. If the patient is male, he may have to have his chest shaved in order to place the electrodes. For both males and females, there may be some discomfort while the electrodes are in place. You should remind patients that during the procedure they should maintain all regular physical activities.

PATIENT EDUCATION AND COMMUNICATION - Pediatric patients require special consideration when explaining the ambulatory monitoring procedure. Consider the child's age and use terms that he or she will understand. To decrease the child's potential anxieties and fears, allow the patient to touch the equipment prior to applying it. Be sure to instruct the parent as well.

Glossary

AC (alternating current) interference - Unwanted markings on the ECG caused by other electrical current sources.

ambulate - To walk.

angina - Pain around the heart radiating to the arm, caused by lack of oxygen to the heart muscle.

angiogram - An invasive procedure during which X-rays are taken of a blood vessel after injection of a radiopaque substance.

angioplasty - Surgical repair of blood vessels.

angle of Louis - A ridge about an inch or so below the suprasternal notch where the main part of the sternum and the top of the sternum, known as the manubrium, are attached.

anterior axillary line - An imaginary vertical line starting at the edge of the chest where the armpit begins.

anti-arrhythmic - Type of medication given to prevent arrhythmias.

aorta - The largest artery of the body, which transports blood from the left ventricle of the heart to the entire body.

aortic semilunar valve - Valve located in the aorta that prevents the backflow of blood into the left ventricle.

apnea - The absence of breathing.

arrhythmia - Abnormal or absence of normal heartbeat, also known as dysrhythmia.

artifact - Unwanted marks on the ECG tracing caused by activity other than the heart's electrical activity.

asystole - When no rhythm or electrical current is traveling through the cardiac conduction system.

atrial kick - When blood is ejected into the ventricles by the atria immediately prior to ventricular systole.

atrioventricular (AV) node - Specialized cells that delay the electrical conduction through the heart and allow the atria time to contract.

atrium (pl. atria) - One of the upper two small chambers of the heart. The right atrium receives blood from the body through the vena cava, and the left atrium receives blood from the lungs through the pulmonary vein.

augmented - Normally small ECG lead tracings that are increased in size by the ECG machine in order to be interpreted.

automaticity - The ability of a cardiac cell to initiate an electrical current to cause a cardiac contraction.

beta blockers - Drugs used to treat hypertension.

bigeminy - Pattern in which every other complex is a premature beat.

biphasic - The waveform has an equally positive (upward) and negative (downward) deflection on the ECG tracing.

bipolar - A type of ECG lead that measures the flow of electrical current in two directions at the same time.

blocked or nonconducted impulse - Impulse occurs too soon after the preceding impulse, causing a period when no other impulses can occur in the ventricles.

bradycardia - A slow heart rate, usually less than 60 beats per minute.

bundle branch block - Impulse is delayed or blocked within the bundle branches of the normal conduction pathway.

bundle branches - Left and right branches of the Bundle of His that conduct impulses down either side of the interventricular septum to the left and right ventricles.

Bundle of His (AV bundle) - A bundle of fibers that originate in the AV node and enter the interventricular septum conducting electrical impulses to the left and right bundle branches.

capture - The ability of the heart muscle to respond to electrical stimulation and depolarize the myocardial tissue.

cardiac cycle - The period from the beginning of one heartbeat to the beginning of the next; the cardiac cycle is made up of the systole and diastole.

cardiac output parameters - Observation guidelines used to assess the blood supply to the vital organs of the body to maintain normal function.

cardiologist - A physician who specializes in the study of the heart.

cardiovascular - Related to the heart and blood vessels (veins and arteries).

Code Blue - The term used for an emergency in a hospital or other health care facility when a person has a cardiac or respiratory arrest.

complex - A group of ECG waveform deflections that indicate electrical activity in the heart.

complexes - Atrial or ventricular contractions as they appear on the ECG; complete ECG waveforms.

conductivity - The ability of the heart cells to receive and transmit an electrical impulse.

congestive heart failure - Failure of the heart to pump an adequate amount of blood to the body tissue.

contractility - The ability of the heart muscle cells to shorten in response to an electrical stimulus.

coronary artery disease - Accumulation of plaque and fatty deposits in the coronary arteries causing a reduction in the blood flow to the heart.

coronary circulation - The circulation of blood to and from the heart muscle.

defibrillator - A machine that produces and sends an electrical shock to the heart, which is intended to correct the electrical pattern of the heart.

deoxygenated blood - Blood that has little or no oxygen (oxygen-poor blood).

depolarization - The electrical activation of the cells of the heart that initiates contraction of the heart muscle.

dextrocardia - An congenital defect (inherited condition) where the left ventricle, left atrium, aortic arch, and stomach are located on the right side of the chest.

diabetes mellitus - (DM) A condition characterized by a lack of production of insulin resulting in elevated glucose (sugar) in the blood stream.

diastole - The phase of the cardiac cycle when the heart is expanding and refilling; also known as the relaxation phase.

echocardiogram - Noninvasive diagnostic test that uses sound to study the heart and blood vessels; also known as an ultrasound.

Einthoven triangle - A triangle formed by three of the limb electrodes—the left arm, the right arm, and the left leg; it is used to determine the first six leads of the 12-lead ECG.

electrocardiogram - A tracing of the heart's electrical activity recorded by an electrocardiograph.

electrocardiograph - An instrument used to record the electrical activity of the heart.

electrocardiology - The study of the heart's electrical activity.

electrodes - Small sensors, metal plates, or disposable units placed on the skin during an ECG to receive the electrical activity from the heart.

excitability - The ability of the heart muscle cells to respond to an impulse or stimulus.

false positive - When a diagnostic test indicates that disease is present but in reality the test is negative and no disease is present.

focus or foci - A cardiac cell or group of cells that function as an ectopic beat.

gain - A control on the ECG machine that increases or decreases the size of the ECG tracing.

galvanometer - An instrument that measures electrical current.

hepatitis - Inflammation of the liver usually caused by a virus.

HIV - (human immunodeficiency virus) The virus that causes AIDS (acquired immune deficiency syndrome).

Holter - Proper name given to one type of ambulatory monitor, named after Norman Holter, inventor of the procedure and machine.

Holter monitor - An instrument that records the electrical activity of the heart during a patient's normal daily activities; also known as an ambulatory monitor.

hypertension - High blood pressure.

hyperventilate - To breathe at an increased rate and depth of inspiration and expiration.

hypotension - Condition in which the patient's blood pressure is not adequate to maintain good blood supply to the vital organs.

inhibited - Electrical current is stopped from being sent to the myocardium.

input - Data entered into an ECG machine, usually through electrodes on the skin surface.

intercostal space (ICS) - The space between two ribs.

interval - The period of time between two activities within the heart.

interventricular septum - A partition or wall that divides the right and left ventricles.

invasive - Procedure that requires entrance into a body cavity, tissue, or blood vessel.

ischemia - Temporary lack of blood supply to an area of tissue due to a blockage in the circulation to that area.

isoelectric - The period when the electrical tracing of the ECG is at zero or a straight line, no positive or negative deflections are seen.

J point - A point on the QRS complex where the depolarization is completed and repolarization starts.

lead - A conductor attached to the ECG machine in the form of a covered wire.

left atrium - The left upper chamber of the heart which receives blood from the lungs.

left ventricle - The left lower chamber of the heart, which pumps oxygenated blood through the body; also known as the workhorse of the heart.

limb - An arm or a leg.

loss of capture - The pacing activity continues to occur without evidence that the electrical activity has depolarized or captured the myocardium.

malfunctioning - The pacemaker fails to send an electrical impulse to the myocardium at the pre-determined interval.

malsensing - The pacemaker does not recognize or sense the patient's own inherent heartbeats.

midaxillary line - An imaginary vertical line that starts at the middle of the armpit.

midclavicular line - An imaginary line on the chest that runs vertically through the center of the clavicle.

mitral (bicuspid) valve - Valve with two cusps or leaflets located between the left atrium and left ventricle; it prevents backflow of blood into the left atrium.

mm (millimeter) - A unit of measurement to indicate time on the ECG tracing. The time is measured on the horizontal axis.

multichannel recorder - An ECG machine that has the ability to record more than one lead tracing at a time, usually 3, 4, or 6.

mV (millivolt) - A unit of measurement to indicate voltage on the ECG tracing. Voltage is measured on the vertical axis.

myocardial - Pertaining to the heart (*cardi*) muscle (*myo*).

myocardial infarction (heart attack) - A blockage of one or more of the coronary arteries causing lack of oxygen to the heart and damage to the muscle tissue.

neurological - Pertaining to the nervous system, its diseases, and its functions.

non-invasive - Procedure that does not require entrance into a body cavity, tissue, or blood vessel.

oscilloscope - A monitor or TV-type device that shows the tracing of the electrical activity of the heart.

output display - The part of the ECG machine that displays the tracing for the electrical activity of the heart, usually in a printed form on a 12-lead ECG machine.

oversensing - The pacemaker senses electrical current from other muscle movements or electrical activity outside of the body as the patient's heart electrical current.

oxygenated blood - Blood having oxygen (oxygen-rich blood).

pacemaker - A cell or group of cells in the heart that affect the rate and rhythm of the heartbeat.

pacemaker (electronic) - A device that delivers a small measured amount of electrical energy to cause myocardial depolarization.

pacemaker competition - Competition between the pacemaker generator and the heart's inherent rate over control of the myocardium.

palpitations - Fast heartbeat sensation felt by the patient, which may or may not be associated with complaints of chest pain.

pericardium - A two-layered sac of tissue enclosing the heart.

polarization - The state of cellular rest in which the inside is negatively charged and the outside is positively charged.

precordial - A type of lead placed on the chest in front of the heart; known as a V lead.

pulmonary artery - Large artery that transports deoxygenated blood from the right ventricle to the lungs. This is the only artery in the body that carries deoxygenated blood.

pulmonary circulation - The transportation of blood to and from the lungs; blood is oxygenated in the lungs during pulmonary circulation.

pulmonary semilunar valve - A valve found in the pulmonary artery that prevents backflow of blood into the right ventricle during pulmonary circulation.

pulmonary vein - A blood vessel that transports blood from the lungs to the left atrium. The only vein in the body to carry oxygenated blood.

Purkinje fibers - The fibers within the heart that distribute electrical impulses from cell to cell throughout the ventricles.

Purkinje network - A network of fibers that distribute electrical impulses through the ventricles; named after a scientist with the last name of Purkinje.

quadgeminy - Pattern in which every fourth complex is a premature beat.

repolarization - When heart muscle cells return to their resting electrical state and the heart muscle relaxes.

rhythm - The regularity of an occurrence such as the heartbeat.

right atrium - The right upper chamber of the heart that receives blood from the body.

right ventricle - The right lower chamber of the heart, which pumps blood to the lungs.

segment - A portion or part of the electrical tracing produced by the heart.

seizure - An interruption of the electrical activity in the brain that causes involuntary muscle movement and sometimes unconsciousness.

semilunar valve - A valve with half-moon-shaped cusps that open and close, allowing blood to travel only one way; located in the pulmonary artery and the aorta.

signal processing - The process within the ECG machine that amplifies the electrical impulse and converts it to a mechanical action on the output display.

single-channel recorder - An ECG machine that records one lead tracing at a time.

sinoatrial (SA) node - An area of specialized cells in the upper right atrium that initiates the heartbeat.

skin rasp - A rough piece of material used to abrade (scrape) the skin prior to electrode placement.

somatic tremor - Voluntary or involuntary muscle movement; also known as body tremor.

speed - A control on the ECG machine that regulates how fast or slow the paper runs during the tracing.

standardization - Setting of the ECG machine output so that 1 millivolt equals 1 centimeter.

stat - Immediately.

stress ECG - Another name for exercise electrocardiography.

stylus - A pointed, penlike instrument that uses heat to record electrical impulse on the ECG graph paper.

suprasternal notch - The dip you feel at the base of the neck just above where the clavicle attaches to the sternum.

supraventricular - An ectopic focus originating above the ventricles, in the atria, or junctional region of the heart.

syncope - Condition when the patient loses consciousness (fainting).

systemic circulation - The circulation between the heart and the entire body, excluding the lungs.

systole - The contraction phase of the cardiac cycle, during which the heart is pumping blood out to the body.

tachycardia - A fast heart rate, usually greater than 100 beats per minute.

target heart rate (THR) - Heart rate measurement needed to truly exercise the heart; determined by 220 minus the patient's age.

technician - An individual who has the knowledge and skills to carry out technical procedures.

technologist - An individual who specializes in a field of science.

telemetry - The transmission of data electronically to an unattached or distant location.

thallium stress test - An invasive type of exercise electrocardiography in which thallium, a radiopaque substance (one that is visible with an X-ray machine), is injected into the body to permit viewing the vessels around the heart.

tricuspid valve - Valve located between the right atrium and right ventricle; it prevents backflow of blood into the right atrium.

trigeminy - Pattern in which every third complex is a premature beat.

triggered - Electrical current is sent from the pacemaker generator to the myocardium to cause the depolarization of the myocardial tissue.

unipolar - A type of ECG lead that measures the flow of electrical current in one direction only.

vagal tone - Condition in which impulses over the vagus nerve exert a continuous inhibitory effect upon the heart, and cause a decrease in heart rate.

vena cava - Largest vein in the body, which provides a pathway for deoxygenated blood to return to the heart; its upper portion, the superior vena cava, transports blood from the head, arms, and upper body, and its lower portion, the inferior vena cava, transports blood from the lower body and legs.

wandering baseline - When the tracing of an ECG drifts away from the center of the paper; also called baseline shift. It has many causes, which can be corrected.

References, Resources, and Further Reading

Adams, Cynthia H., and Peter D. Jones, *Interpersonal Skills and Health Professional Issues,* Glencoe/McGraw-Hill, Peoria, IL, 2001.

Aehlert, Barbara, *ECGs Made Easy,* Mosby, St. Louis, MO, 1995.

Cohn, Elizabeth Gross, and Mary Gilroy-Doohan, *Flip and See ECG,* W.B. Saunders Co., Philadelphia, PA, 1996.

Garrison, *Introduction to Human Relations,* Glencoe/McGraw-Hill, Westerville, OH, 1995.

Haddix, Kathryn A., *ECG Basics, Total Care Programming,* Richmond, VA, 1998.

————, *Infection Control for Health Care and Nursing CD-ROM software,* Total Care Programming, Richmond, VA, 1997.

Judson, Karen, and Sharon Blesie Hicks, *Glencoe Law and Ethics for Medical Careers,* Glencoe/McGraw-Hill, Second Edition, Westerville, OH, 1999.

Lamberton, Lowell, *Human Relations: Strategies for Success,* Glencoe/McGraw-Hill, Westerville, OH, 1995.

Makely, Sherry, *Multiskilled Health Care Workers: Issues and Approaches to Cross-Training,* Pine Ridge Publications, Inc., Bloomington, IN, 1998.

Minor-Evans, Leslie, and Lowell Lamberton, *Working with People: A Human Relations Guide,* Glencoe/McGraw-Hill, Westerville, OH, 1997.

Prickett-Ramutkowsski et al., *Glencoe Clinical Procedures for Medical Assisting,* Glencoe/McGraw-Hill, Westerville, OH, 1999.

Thaler, Malcolm S., *The Only EKG Book You'll Ever Need,* J.B. Lippincott Co., Philadelphia, PA, 1996.

Wiederhold, Richard, *Electrocardiography: The Monitoring Lead,* W.B. Saunders Co., Philadelphia, PA, 1988.

Index